Medical Humanities Companion

VOLUME THREE

Medical Humanities Companion

VOLUME THREE

Treatment

Edited by
Pekka Louhiala
Iona Heath
and
John Saunders

Radcliffe Publishing
Oxford • New York

Radcliffe Publishing Ltd
St Mark's House
Shepherdess Walk
London
N1 7LH
United Kingdom

www.radcliffehealth.com

Electronic catalogue and worldwide online ordering facility.

British Library Cataloguing in Publication Data

A catalogue record for this book is available from the British Library.

ISBN-13: 978 184619 370 5

Typeset by Phoenix Photosetting, Chatham, Kent, UK
Printed and bound by Cadmus Communications, USA

Contents

About the editors and authors

Rolf Ahlzén is a general practitioner and an assistant professor in medical humanities at Karlstad University in Sweden. He has an academic background both in the humanities and in medicine, and he is the chairman of the Regional Ethical Committee.

Martyn Evans joined Durham University in 2002 as Professor of Humanities in Medicine and Principal of John Snow College, and he became Principal of Trevelyan College in 2008. He taught philosophy and ethics of medicine at the University of Wales for several years. He was founding joint editor of the *Medical Humanities* edition of the *Journal of Medical Ethics* from 2000 to 2008. He has published variously on the aesthetics of music, ethics and philosophy of medicine, and the role of humanities in medical education. His current interests include music and medicine, the philosophy of wonder and philosophical problems in medicine. In 2005 he was made an honorary Fellow of the Royal College of General Practitioners.

Jill Gordon is a general practitioner specialising in psychotherapy in primary care in Sydney. She is President of the Australian College of Psychological Medicine and an honorary professor at the University of Sydney where she initiated Australia's first postgraduate degree in medical humanities.

Iona Heath worked as a GP in Kentish Town in London from 1975 to 2010. She was President of the Royal College of General Practitioners, UK, from 2009 to 2012.

Pekka Louhiala is a lecturer in medical ethics at the University of Helsinki, Finland. He has degrees in both medicine and philosophy, and he also works as a part-time paediatrician in private practice. He has published on various topics in medical ethics, philosophy of medicine and epidemiology. His current academic interests include conceptual and philosophical issues in medicine, such as evidence-based medicine and placebo effects.

Anne Macleod, poet and novelist, was formerly Associate Specialist in Dermatology at Aberdeen Royal Infirmary.

Jane Macnaughton is Professor of Medical Humanities and Co-Director of the Centre for Medical Humanities at Durham University. She is also Deputy Head of the University's School of Medicine and Health and teaches on its undergraduate medical programme. She has published on a wide range of themes within the medical humanities, including the doctor–patient relationship, embodied practice, medical education and the role of medical humanities in critiquing the evidence-base of biomedicine. Having worked as a GP before moving to full time academic work in Durham, Jane now does part-time clinical work in gynaecology and is Honorary Consultant in Obstetrics and Gynaecology at the University Hospital of North Durham.

Raimo Puustinen is a general practitioner with 30 years of clinical experience. He currently works as an acting professor of General Practice at the University of Tampere Medical School, Finland. He has published articles and books on general practice, medical ethics and philosophy of medicine. When not practising medicine or contemplating theoretical issues in medical practice, he plays jazz on the tenor saxophone and blues with a blues harp. He is married, and has four children and six grandchildren.

Carl Edvard Rudebeck is a general practitioner from Västervik in Sweden. He is a research advisor in the healthcare organisation of Kalmar county, and part-time professor of general practice at Tromsö University in Norway. He is involved in various qualitative research projects in general practice and physiotherapy. He has put much interest into the theoretical aspects of general practice as a discipline, and into the phenomenology of body experience and the phenomenology of the doctor–patient interaction.

John Saunders is a consultant physician in Abergavenny, South Wales; honorary professor at Swansea University; former visiting professor at the University of Otago, New Zealand; and honorary senior lecturer at Cardiff University. He was formerly an associate editor of *Medical Humanities*, chair of the Research Ethics Committee for Wales; and is current chair of ethics at the Royal College of Physicians. He recently completed postgraduate studies in philosophy at University College London.

Introduction

Symptom leads to diagnosis; diagnosis leads to treatment. That may be a simple viewpoint for the everyday experience of the average patient. Treatment is an active process: in treatment, somebody does something. The outcome may then be related to that something. Of course it may not: treatment may be ineffective, inappropriate or inadequate. In the first volume of this series, we emphasised the subjectivities that patients bring to their symptom experience. Diagnosis, which we explored in the second volume, turned out to be rather more than the objective process that is so often presented to practitioners in training. Treatment has always lacked such objectivities. Entire systems of treatment have competed with one another over centuries and the triumph of scientific medicine has not been total. Competing systems continue to make their contribution as alternatives or as adjuncts. As Thomas points out, 'If magic is to be defined as the employment of ineffective techniques to allay anxiety when effective ones are not available, then we must recognise that no society will ever be free from it.'[1] But even within the box labelled 'scientific', there is a great deal more to be said than the facts of Mr Gradgrind.[2] Sometimes patients do better with treatments that they believe in; sometimes their confidence in the efficacy of a treatment makes no difference at all. Sometimes treatments are imposed: notably to the non-autonomous patient, where there is no other option, but also resulting from the advice of the professional practitioner. Where are these boundaries to be drawn? How much can be demanded in a healthcare system necessarily limited in its resources and where the price of choice for one may be the restriction of service for the other? Added to these practical ethical concerns are the underlying issues of belief about efficacy, the meaning of treatment in the patient's overall life experience, the significance of treatment for those who have no identifiable malady and the supposed contrasts between caring and curing.

In this volume we continue to follow the fortunes of our fictionalised patients as they undergo the therapeutic experience. If scientific medicine is grounded in the general, one strong contribution from the humanities is to study the application of that knowledge to concrete human beings in all their diversity, difference and individuality. The outcome of those considerations is to realise the human dimension of care in daily practice. Once again we invite our readers to accompany our 'patients' – and us – as we continue our journeys.

Pekka Louhiala, Iona Heath and John Saunders
June 2013

REFERENCES

1 Thomas K. *Religion and the Decline of Magic*. London: Weidenfeld & Nicholson; 1971. p. 800.
2 Dickens C. *Hard Times*. London: Chapman & Hall; 1854. Mr Thomas Gradgrind is a schoolmaster who opens Dickens's novel with his declaration on the 'One Thing Needful' saying, '[W]hat I want is Facts. Teach these boys and girls nothing but Facts. Facts alone are wanted in life.'

Acknowledgement

We wish to acknowledge Glenn Colquhoun, doctor and poet from New Zealand, for kind permission to use his poem *Playing God*.

Playing God

She asked me if she took one pill for her
heart and one pill for her hips and one pill
for her chest and one pill for her blood
how come they would all know which part
of her body they should go to.

I explained to her that active metabolites in each
pharmaceutical would adopt a spatial configuration
leading to an exact interface with receptor molecules
on the cellular surfaces of the target structures involved.

She told me not to bullshit her.

I told her each pill had a different shape and that
each part of her body had a different shape and that
her pills could only work when both of these shapes could
fit together.

She said I had no right to talk about the shape of her body.

I said that each pill was a key and that her body was
ten thousand locks.

She said she wasn't going to swallow that.

I told her they worked by magic.

She asked me why I didn't say that in the first place.

GLENN COLQUHOUN

The patients' stories

ANNE MACLEOD

RACHEL

When we go to the hospital, Mum looks nervous. It's like she's back at school, about to do a test. She puts on her best clothes and takes her best handbag and sits in the waiting room, stiff as a wooden chair. I always take a book. If I fidget at all, she glowers at me as if we were in church.

We usually see Dax, the diabetic nurse, and then one of the doctors. Not always the same one. I think that's what sets Mum off – why she gets in such a panic – and why she wants my sugar levels to be as good as they can be. If it weren't for Dax, I don't know what we'd do. Mum phones her all the time, always checking. If it were me, I'd be driven daft. Dax never seems to mind.

'That's what I'm here for, Mrs Walcott,' she always says. 'Phone any time you like.'

It was Dax who taught me how to poke my finger with the lancet, and squeeze my finger to make the little drop of blood for the meter. She showed me how to hold the test strip carefully against the small round drop so that it would fill up properly. She taught me how to read the result, how to use an insulin pen and all about carb counting.

Back at the start, I couldn't take it all in – and Mum still can't – but Dax keeps trying. Like Auntie Vimal across the street. (She's not my real auntie, but I've known her all my life. You should see her saris – beautiful. Sometimes she lets me play with them.) Auntie Vimal's sister has diabetes, too.

'It never held her back. She's married now with two fine children of her own!' Auntie Vimal always says that. Auntie Vimal was a nurse. If Mum isn't on the phone to Dax, she's over the road at Auntie Vimal's.

I don't know why Mum's such a wimp at the clinic. With the doctors she pretends to know it all and they seem to believe her. It's Dax who has to ask the questions for us; it's Dax who really knows how things have been. It's Dax who sorts things out. When she can.

Dax went ballistic when the school wouldn't let me go on my class trip to Alton Towers. I went ballistic, too. See, Mrs Schneider stopped me after school, holding me back after the others to give me the news.

'I realise you'll be a little disappointed,' she had said with a smile. 'But it's for the best. We have to keep things safe.'

She wanted me to smile and say, 'That's fine.' But I'd been looking forward to that trip all year. I couldn't wait for the whole class to be away together staying in a hostel and – best of all – the rides! Leroy had looked them up on the computer for me. I burst into tears. I screamed like a baby.

Dax helped Mum write a letter to Mrs Schneider. When that made no difference, Dax phoned the Head. Didn't get anywhere.

'I'm sorry, Rachel.' She sighed. 'I'll ask Dr Friend to write.'

But Dr Friend was away that week. By the time his letter reached the school it was too late. The trip was over. So Dax helped Mum fill out an application to Diabetes UK for me to attend one of their Children's Holidays at this centre near Northampton. A Frontier Centre. I can't wait.

I don't like having diabetes. I don't like the finger poking and injecting, although you do get used to it. I don't like Mum being worried all the time. (Dax says she will relax. Eventually.) But Leroy? He's been cool – looked on YouTube and found me lots of kids' *own* home-made films about their diabetes and how they live with it.

Like *Diabetes Angels*.

One of the kids in that film looks a bit like me: brown skin, dark braids and a broad yellow hairband. She lives in America. She won't be at Northampton, but there will be lots of kids exactly like me. At Frontier Camp I'll have a lot of fun and I'll be ordinary.

Believe me, that will be the best thing of all.

JAKE

When Jake opened the kitchen door, he knew the game was up. Carol sat at the table. The angle of her head and the way that her hair swung impatiently about her shoulders told its own story. In her hand was a manilla envelope. She tapped the table with it, an angry staccato rhythm.

Jake tried to bluster through, dredged up a smile, setting two plastic bags of shopping on the floor.

'You're early. I wasn't expecting you so soon … '

'Clearly.' The tone was dry.

'Did you catch an early train?'

'Don't try to change the subject.' She flung the opened letter across the table. 'Your hospital appointment.' Colour flooded Jake's cheeks. He could feel the stiffening hunch of his shoulders. Said nothing. There was nothing he could say. 'Your appointment was *three* months ago. When you didn't turn up, they sent another – and then another –' Jake stared at the floor. 'This letter is a copy of the note they wrote your GP telling her they won't send for you again.' She waved it at him. 'What were you thinking of, Jake? You'll have to phone the hospital. Apologise. Get this sorted.'

'No.'

'What do you mean, *no*?'

'I'm not going, Carol. I don't want any more tubes stuck up and through me. I'm not a *freak*.'

'No one said you were. Don't be so feeble. It isn't all that bad.'

'How would you know? You aren't the one who has to go through it. I don't want any more of those bloody tests and I don't want any bloody pills either.'

'But Jake—'

'That's final, Carol. I can't do it. You saw how it was that time I went to the surgery. I won't let them touch me again. It's *my* choice. It's my body.'

'And what about the pain? The diarrhoea? What about all those nights you spend in agony?'

'You're at college in Bristol! What would you know about it? One visit in four months!' He swallowed and looked away. 'I may not be at college, but I can guess what's coming next – the old *let's-just-be-friends*. Got it in one there, didn't I? And you think that gives you the right to swan in here and read my mail? For any's sake!'

'Jake—'

'Leave it, Carol! Leave me alone! OK? '

The kitchen door and flat door slammed in sequence. Carol stayed at the table, shivering. She heard Jake crashing down the stairs and out on to the street. She sighed and picked up the letter, blinking. Tears were not far away.

Jake ran blindly along the streets, ran and ran and ran, splashing through the downpour. Sharp, stinging drops sliced into his hair and clothes, like a thousand needles, like Carol's words.

He meant what he said. He wasn't going back, not for more of that. What did she know about it? What did she care? Who was she to judge? Besides, the peppermint oil did help a bit when he took it. Things were not so bad. Not like they had been. And as for Carol? He'd get over her. Should have seen it coming.

At this thought, colic flickered through his gut. A warning. Jake stopped running, bent double. 'Noo—' The cramping escalated, hot and white. Pain grew and grew – plateaued for an instant – and then cut deep into him like a knife, twisting and spiralling.

Jake closed his eyes. Couldn't move. He'd need to find a toilet, but where? Where was he anyway?

'What is it, boy?' The voice was female, old and frail. 'Lad, do you need help? Are you OK?'

LIZ

Dr Wocjik had warned Liz to take the day off work.

'You'll want to take it easy. Give yourself time. Ask a friend to go with you.'

Dr Wocjik was being her usual social self. Liz smiled and did not say how impossible she found it to discuss intimate problems like this. *Who was there anyway? Her mother? Not a chance.* Her mother was the last person in the world with whom she could or would have broached the subject. Nor was it easy persuading Dave to leave that Monday free; it was the busiest day of the week in the agency.

'Must it be Monday? Carla's off. We're under pressure on the Maitland contract as it is. '

'I'll have everything in order by Friday. No problem, Dave. Any last minute changes can be layered in. You're the world's expert on that.'

'Not with old man Maitland. He needs the female touch. You and Carla can wind him round your little fingers, whereas I—'

'Dave, you know how hard it is to find an NHS dentist – root canal treatment – I won't exactly be enjoying it—' Liz did not like lying. It would have been simpler to tell the truth but she could not bring herself to do that. Dave shook his head and shrugged. 'You're an angel, Dave. I'll do the same for you.'

Sophie's school had chosen the same Monday to stage their parents' evening. She would surely manage that.

She said nothing to Sophie as she left her at the school gate. Later, in the waiting room, thoughts she'd been struggling to hold at bay swept in, restless as a sharp spring tide, casting her adrift. Her first smear had been scant. The second – so the letter said – showed abnormalities. Dr Wocjik had explained.

'CIN2. That's moderate untidiness. *Not* cancer. But it needs in-depth assessment, Liz. And treatment.'

Hence her attendance at this clinic for colposcopy. An abnormal smear could and did – for some women – mean cancer. Was that why the clinic had been painted pastel pink, and why the nurses and receptionists were decked in lavender and the baby blue? Despite the colour scheme, and despite the relentlessly bland background music, none of the women waiting on these tasteful chairs looked comfortable. None of them looked anything but anxious.

The waiting room was full.

Liz tried to settle down and read but the book she'd picked up in the station – a story of three women setting out to find as many sexual partners as they could – did not, in the circumstances, seem light or comforting. She glanced at her appointment letter again.

'Mrs Diaz?' Liz looked up, surprised to have been taken on time, given the press of women on the pastel chairs. She followed the nurse along a maze of corridors, the nurse talking as they went. Liz struggled to keep up.

'Dr Patience is looking after you today,' the nurse rambled. 'With three fifth-year students. She will introduce them to you.' Liz stopped dead. Shook her head.

'I don't want any students.' The nurse looked confused.

'We are a teaching hospital,' she said finally. 'Everyone has to learn.'

'No students,' Liz insisted.

'I'll speak to the doctor. Wait here.' She abandoned Liz in the corridor, sweeping into a clinic room. The door closed firmly behind her.

Things went from bad to worse after that. Liz waited forlornly in the corridor as three white-coated figures shuffled from the room. She felt a little embarrassed as they passed; they were all ridiculously young-looking – a girl wearing a veil, a six-foot youngster with a shock of red, untidy hair and a thin Chinese-looking girl who may have been Malaysian. *They did not,* Liz thought, *seem particularly downcast.* It was, she reminded herself, her right to ask for privacy. But the nurse looked at her coldly, and the eponymous Dr Patience did not live up to her name. Instructions and explanations were delivered in what seemed to Liz to be a brusque and perfunctory manner, although she did, it must be said, talk Liz through the procedure. She warned her that her feet would be in stirrups, explained the insertion of the speculum, and the examination with the colposcope itself – a somewhat alarming instrument that seemed to Liz like a microscope bearing down towards her starkly exposed lower end. Liz turned down the offer of seeing for herself the results of the examination on the TV screen to her right. Did some women actually want to *watch*?

'I'm going to wash the cervix with a little acetic acid,' Dr Patience intoned. 'That will help display any abnormality. You should feel very little. Most women find it simple.' Liz struggled to remain calm and relaxed. She was not calm. She was not relaxed.

'Mrs Diaz.' Dr Patience stretched towards a trolley beside her. She did not meet Liz's eye.

'There is a little evidence here of abnormality at the mouth of the cervix, a small patch of tissue that we can remove for you today. Easiest to get it over and done with, no?' She nodded to the nurse who bustled around the room, fiddling with things Liz could not see. 'We call this a LLETZ,' the doctor continued. 'Just a small shot of local anaesthetic now – you won't feel a thing.' A sticky electrode was slapped on her thigh. Liz jumped.

'What's happening?'

'We use an electric loop to take the sample. It cuts and seals the tissue at the one time. Both investigates and treats. Now, relax. The worst is over.' It wasn't.

The doctor introduced an instrument that Liz couldn't see into the speculum. Liz twitched involuntarily, groaning at a sharp pain – like period pain but harsher. There was, too, a sense of heat, and the smell of burning flesh. This smell was the worst thing of all.

'Try to keep still,' Dr Patience advised. Liz found it difficult.

'Ooh—'

'Good.' Dr Patience kept working. 'Nearly there – good, that's it now. There. The sample takes six weeks at least to process. We should have got it all, but the lab will let us know.

'This treatment is all that's needed in 95 to 98 out of 100 cases, which leaves a 1 in 20 or 1 in 50 chance of failure. It doesn't affect future fertility. Don't go worrying about that.

'We'll see you again in four months, and then six months after. You'll need repeat smears annually for a time.'

'Every year?'

'For at least the next five years. Perhaps ten. Any questions?'

'It's still very sore,' Liz complained. 'Is that normal?' The doctor shook her head. Looked at the screen.

'Unusual. The cervix looks OK. No bleeding at all. Nor is it burdened with too many nerve endings. Try to relax. I'll slip this out. That's good.' She withdrew the speculum.

But salt saliva welled in Liz's mouth. The sterile clinic room was swimming around her.

'Nurse,' Dr Patience's voice now held an edge of urgency. 'Nurse, lower the table head.' Liz felt sweaty and sick. 'Get her feet down.' Liz felt her legs being lifted from the stirrups and set back on the trolley, which had magically grown a lower end. 'Pulse fine. Check the blood pressure.'

Dr Patience turned away, leaving Liz to the nurse's flurried ministrations.

Back in the pastel waiting room, half an hour later, Liz sipped a mug of hot sweet tea. A simple faint, they'd said. It happened.

'If you need another LLETZ,' had been the doctor's parting shot, 'perhaps you would consider a general.' Which general? Liz smiled, weakly. Mark Anthony? Napoleon? Alexander the Great? Napoleon would at least be good in bed.

'Is there a Mrs Diaz?' a receptionist interrupted. 'One last call—' she raised her voice. 'Taxi for Diaz—'

GEOFF

Jane shut the car door and waited for Jen to ease herself out of the passenger seat. It took her sister an age to do this. She rose to unsteady feet. Jen waited, clicking the electronic lock.

'Where do we go from here?'

'This way.' Jen nodded. 'Hope Ward, it's called.'

'As in *Abandon hope, all ye who enter here*?' Jane frowned at the brick-built walls. 'Cheerful.'

Jen clucked. 'It's called Hope Ward after Bob Hope. He visited back in the 40s. During the war this hospital was full of GIs.'

'Oversexed, overpaid and over here?'

Already out of breath, Jen did not answer. Jane was forced to wait at the top of the steps for her increasingly emaciated twin. She tried to smile and look cheerful, so as not to let her expression give her away. It had been hard to keep her spirits up since that last phone call when Jen had told her everything. About her own lung cancer, Geoff's depression, how Mary could not cope and how he had been admitted to hospital.

'He's not that great.' Jen wheezed. 'These things take time.'

Looking at her sister – so thin you'd almost swear you could see through her – Jane wondered how much time they had. 'Take my arm,' she told her. 'Lean on me.' Her sister was no weight at all.

'Mark flew over last week.'

'Good. And Mary?'

Jen shook her head. 'Mary's too upset to come.'

'She put him in.'

Jen changed the subject. 'This way, Jane. This door here—'

Geoff was in a single room, not far from the ward entrance. Jane, despite herself, was not unimpressed. Although the walls were white, the room was not too clinical. The duvet cover and curtains – both red and green – were floral. A small television screen hung in a corner opposite the bed, next to the en-suite shower and toilet. The view from the window, currently in full sun, was of the neat herb garden, beside which they'd parked.

'Geoff!' She held her hand out. 'Great to see you. Feeling any better?' Geoff stared past her. He sat in the armchair beside the bed, a tartan rug across his knees.

'How are you, my dear?' asked Jen. 'Did you have a good night? Look who has come all the way from Reading, just for you—'

'Good afternoon, Mrs Doughty.' A young nurse swung into the room. 'Sister would like you to call in at her office on your way out.' She stopped, uncertain, her eyes swinging from Jen to Jane, Jane to Jen.

'Goodness – you must be –'

'Twins,' Jane pre-empted her. 'Even our names are identical. I'm Jane. She's Jen – Jennifer. Our parents should have had more sense. Where will we find this office?'

'Beside the nursing station.'

'Thanks. See you shortly.'

The nurse wrote something on a chart at the foot of Geoff's bed, and stooped to reach his buzzer, which had fallen on the floor. She tucked this on the chair beside him. 'There you go. See you later, Geoff. I'll do your observations then. Anything you're needing? No?'

Jane turned her attention back to Jen, who was sitting on the bed beside her husband, stroking his hand, murmuring about the garden: which plants were flourishing, which were in bud and which needed attention. Geoff stared resolutely out of the window and did not look or speak – not once – throughout the full half hour they sat there.

'Geoff,' Jane interrupted at last. 'You look tired. We should be going.' Jen nodded, but did not release his hand.

'We'll come back tomorrow, Geoff, after lunch.' Even to Jane's own ears, her voice sounded too bright. Artificial. As they left the room, she thought she caught a flicker of movement in Geoff's eyes – a glint of tears. Confusion.

'Let's find this office and then get home. I need a cup of tea.'

She walked at the slow pace that Jen could almost manage.

Sister Merchant looked young – no more than 30. Her room was cramped and windowless; a large computer desk left room for little else. Two plastic chairs had been squeezed in beside the door. 'Please sit down.' She started talking before they had settled themselves. 'Mr Doughty,' she began, 'is making progress. You will have seen a change these last few days, a lightening of mood. The antidepressants are beginning to work, and the physiotherapist is pleased with him, too. We wondered if this may not be the time to begin to think about discharge plans.'

Jane was confused. *Discharge?*

'I know you were his carer and your daughter has told us how well you managed. But it sounds as though extra help may now be needed. Mr Doughty's admission was precipitated, I think, by a spell of illness of your own. What we need to do is assess the situation. If all is now well and you are comfortable with the notion of taking Mr Doughty home and managing as before – *if* you are confident – then we can set up a simple discharge, and we need not involve the Social Work Department. However, if you need extra help, Social Work review would be a good idea.'

'Not Social Work,' said Jen. 'Wouldn't that slow things up terribly? Can't I just take him home?'

Jane could not believe her ears. 'Sister,' she said, 'we need to talk. Jen, why don't you go back and spend a few more minutes with Geoff? Come on, I'll take you.' She nodded at Sister Merchant. 'I'll be back.'

'I can find my own way—'

Jen's protest was ignored. Jane walked slowly back along the corridor beside her.

'What on earth are you trying to do? Where's your head in all this? Look at you. You can hardly hold yourself up. You don't even drive. How would you manage Geoff?' Jen shrugged, despondent. 'He's a lot of work,' Jane insisted. 'Needs so much – everything – done for him. You can't take that responsibility right now, Jen. You're not fit. Don't even know the plan for your own treatment. Do you?' Jen shook her head. 'When are you seeing the consultant?'

'Wednesday. But it's not TB, Jen. Dr Murray said so.' Jane sighed. They'd been round this one before.

'Jen, you must be sensible. You can't take Geoff home until you're able to cope. We don't know yet when that day will be.' *Or if that day will be,* Jane thought. 'Yes, he feels the separation. So must you. It won't be for ever. Go on, sit with him. Talk to him. I'll bring Sister Merchant up to date. You can't make any plans today.'

Geoff's eyes brightened – clearly brightened – as Jen entered the room and sat herself beside him, clasping his good hand. Jane shut the door quietly and retraced her steps.

She would have to make plans herself. *What would they do if Jen was as ill as she looked? How could they look after her? And Geoff? No one could manage him like Jen. They were a closed unit. No one else mattered, not to them. That was why Mary's anger at Jen was from the first, so bitter. The girl felt – always had – shut out. Unneeded. And they didn't see it. Couldn't help themselves. With Jen and Geoff it always had been true love. Unmitigated.*

JEN

Dr Murray's kind face was the only thing Jen remembered afterwards. His words – most of his words – were gone. *How could that be?* He spent half an hour with her and he did most of the talking. His face made her think of the actor who played the head of MI5 in a television programme years ago. The kind of face that would have gone with a powdered wig and patch, although Dr Murray was clearly a very modern doctor.

'I want you to speak to our Macmillan nurse,' Dr Murray said. 'She'll go over it all again. Have you any questions about the condition, or the treatment? If you think of anything – anything at all – don't be afraid to come back and ask.'

Jen's mind was blank. It may, after all, have been a good idea to allow Jane to come with her. She had refused, had turned down even the option of a lift to the hospital.

'Stubborn.' Jane sighed.

That was true. Jen was stubborn. She always had been.

The nurse made her a cup of tea and explained again about her diagnosis. Small-cell cancer, which meant the best treatment was chemotherapy. She glossed over the details. Jen didn't push for more information.' Some people call it oat-cell,' the nurse informed, 'because of how it looks down the microscope.'

'Like porridge,' said Jen, oddly entranced.

The nurse smiled. 'Not exactly.'

But from that moment on, Jen thought of the tumour as porridge – and she thought of the chemotherapy as milk struggling to dissipate the conglomeration.

She went back into hospital for chemotherapy, the day after the clinic visit. The same ward she'd had the tests in, but they gave her a room to herself this time, and the drip meant she was more or less confined to the bed. Each time the nurses came, they took great care to double- and triple-check the drugs. That surprised Jen. Nurses were always careful, but to see them so focused made her realise, as nothing had, that the treatment was serious. Cancer was serious. *It was not TB and you could treat it, but at what cost?*

When Margaret, the Macmillan nurse, fitted her for a wig, Jen cried.

'Sorry. Didn't mean to do that. It's just—'

'Your hair will grow back.' Margaret's tone was reassuring. 'But wigs are really great these days, so natural. If we get it all arranged and measured at this stage you'll have it when you need it.'

Jen thought of the day she had met Geoff – before his wife was ill. He was married.

So was she. Geoff stared at her swinging chestnut bob; he could not take his eyes off what she knew was her best asset. She strolled across Station Square relishing the feeling that Geoff Doughty, the best-looking man in the bus company, obviously fancied her. She worked with another driver, and she saw Geoff hardly at all, but every time she did she knew he really liked what he saw.

What will he think when he sees she has no hair?

The chemo was not easy. Jen vomited and had diarrhoea so sudden and excessive that she couldn't make it to the bathroom and fouled the bed. The nurses didn't seem to mind. Jen couldn't stand the smell.

'We've seen it all – that's what we're here for.'

Nobody had warned her it could happen. Jen felt humiliated. Her body letting her down. Like Geoff's.

'It happens,' said the nurse.

'I hope not,' Jen said. 'How many times do I have to do this? How will I ever cope?'

It was amazing, however, what she did cope with.

Tiredness. Fatigue. She was so glad that Jane was able to spend a few weeks with her. Mark, her son in New York, could not have come. Mary, Geoff's daughter, did not come – did not even send a card. Jen did not expect it.

The worst thing was the mouth ulcers. So painful. She didn't feel like food, but if she had she would have found it impossible to eat. Even drinking was difficult – the smallest drop an achievement. The mouthwash seemed to make things worse.

Then there were the blood tests. They went on for ever. Her results were so bad that they wouldn't let her visit Geoff, who must be wondering where she was. He didn't know about the cancer. She wouldn't let Jane tell him.

I'll tell him my own way, in my own time.

She worried about him. *Was he eating? Was he lonely?* When Jane came back and told her that they'd put him in a ward with other men, she fretted. *He'd always been a private man. How would he cope with the lack of privacy?* 'It's fine,' said Jane. 'He seems to like the company.'

The nausea settled, but Jen woke up one morning to find her hair lying on the pillow. The wig had not arrived. Jane wrapped a green scarf around her head.

'Perfect for the land army!'

Jen had stopped looking in her mirror.

'Land army?' She tried to smile. 'No, that's a different war. Do you think Geoff will mind?'

'He'll never notice.'

Jane didn't mean to hurt her, but this, more than anything, terrified Jen and made her cry.

What if she died? Would he notice then?

1

On treatment and its effects

JANE MACNAUGHTON

I did not imagine being bald at forty four.[1]

This book is about treatment and what it does to people – patients, doctors and relatives – and to their relationships and wider lives. Treatment has, at times, as Julia Darling observes in her poem 'Chemotherapy' (quoted from above), unimaginable effects on us: on our bodies, but also on how we live and understand ourselves in the context of our lives. For doctors to treat well it is important to realise that treatment can lead to patients feeling confused, distressed and dislodged from their lives not just by the physical changes brought about by treatment but also by how it changes their understanding of their bodies. It is not possible for doctors to anticipate all of the possible changes that episodes of treatment may bring about for patients, but this chapter aims to explore some of the ways that those changes may be experienced by patients.

Treating others well is important: we all aspire to do this in our lives. What is distinctive about treating in a medical context?

SENSES OF 'TREATMENT'

'Treatment' is an extraordinarily malleable word in the English language. Depending on its context it has a number of different meanings, connotations and feelings associated with it. With children we talk of 'treats' and 'treating' as fun events on birthdays and holidays, something to look forward to that has been arranged for their pleasure. This meaning seems to have little resonance with the clinical context, as few patients would regard the visit to the doctor as a treat in this sense! The way we 'treat' people speaks of our approach to others and normally carries a moral connotation: that we treat them either well or badly. This everyday sense does have a relationship with the clinical idea of treatment, as the 'treatment' (noun) is part of the interaction between patient and doctor; it is part of the way that the doctor treats the patient. Some medical educators would say that treatment starts the minute that the patient walks through the door, in that the way in which the doctor shows interest, asks questions and listens can have profound effects on the responsiveness of patients to the more formal measures that clinicians take to deal with the diagnosed problem, as Michael Balint explored as long ago as the 1950s.[2] We will be discussing this issue in more detail in Chapter 6.

There is a further sense of 'treat' in the academic context meaning how a subject is examined or alluded to in literature or art. For example, the subject of Christ and his relationship to his mother Mary is given a range of different 'treatments' in art, thus allowing critics to reflect upon the cultural context and perspective of the artists and viewers of the day. This interesting sense may tangentially throw some light upon our understanding of the notion in its clinical context. The doctor's treatment of the patient, as well as revealing her abilities in communication and her clinical knowledge and skills, also exposes her idea of the patient as a 'patient'. The way that she 'treats of' the patient (in literary critical language) may undergo a subtle change as her conclusion about diagnosis begins to firm in her mind. As certain viewpoints become closed off and as the direction and context become clearer as she decides what to do the change can communicate itself to the patient in subtle ways. If the treatment is something that the doctor needs to hand on to a specialist colleague, for example, referral may lead to a suspension of attention from the GP while the consultant takes over the patient's care. As the diagnosis firms up and treatment gets underway, the patient can find herself categorised and contained: 'The lung cancer having chemotherapy in bed ten (Jen)'; 'The next patient is a LLETZ biopsy (Liz).'

These senses do not just remind us of dictionary definitions but of the importance of words and the impact that they can have through the range and subtleties of meaning they can hold at one and the same time. The theme of this book takes us to what for many patients and doctors is the nub of medicine: how doctors try to make patients better. It is a high-stakes aspect of the clinical interaction and, as such, holds greater potential for problems, pitfalls and misunderstandings than any other. Therefore, these nuances of meaning are important, and we need to hold them in our minds and think of the way they inform the notion of treatment as it is understood and lived by both doctors and patients.

WHAT IS 'TREATMENT'?

In the clinical context, then, what is 'treatment'? Treatment is conventionally understood to be something that the doctor does to or provides for the patient in order to cure or alleviate the problem that he or she has presented. That may be a surgical operation (such as the large loop excision of the transformation zone (LLETZ) experienced by Liz) or it may be the administration of a drug by injection (such as Rachel's insulin) or by mouth. Conventionally also, the doctor is the one who understands the nature of the treatment and its effects; and, although she may explain these to the patient, much is still taken on the patient's part on trust as the detailed implications and interactions are the subject of many years of study and expertise. The doctor may explain what it is that is going to happen but that does not mean that the patient is prepared or that he or she understands these implications. Understanding what is happening involves a cognitive grasp of the series of events that make up the treatment episode. For two of our patients, Liz and Jen (both of whose treatment is described in some detail), the series of events is clear. For Liz, she is examined, injected with local anaesthetic, has a small piece of cervix removed, feels dizzy and faints. For Jen, she has a drip put up while she is in bed, a number of packs of drugs are run through the drip, she vomits and is incontinent and suffers fatigue and hair loss. These spare accounts of the treatment episodes are common to the understanding of both doctor and patient involved (although one may argue that Liz is not fully aware of what is happening to her); however, it is obvious that the perceptions of doctor and patient of the treatment event are very different.

Consider these two very different accounts of the side effects of treatment for breast cancer.

From the *New England Journal of Medicine* (*NEJM*) 'Side effects of adjuvant treatment of breast cancer':

> There are several problems in identifying and estimating the frequency of treatment-related side effects. Information about side effects is often derived from retrospective case-control and registry studies that have been subject to several biases. Some treatment-related side effects resemble diseases prevalent in older women. The effects of radiation or anthracyclines [class of drugs used in cancer chemotherapy] on the heart may be difficult to detect, given the increasing rates of cardiovascular disease as women age. The most reliable information about side effects comes from clinical trials conducted decades ago.
>
> Many women with breast cancer who are receiving adjuvant chemotherapy have fatigue, and about two thirds of them rate the level of fatigue as moderate or severe. .... The fatigue appears to resolve after treatment. In a survey of nearly 2000 women with breast cancer who were evaluated three years after adjuvant treatment, the level of fatigue was similar to that of age-matched women.[3]

From Julia Darling's 'Chemotherapy' in *Sudden Collapses in Public Places*:

> I did not imagine being bald
> at forty four. I didn't have a plan.
> Perhaps a scar or two from growing old,
> Hot flushes. I'd sit fluttering a fan.
>
> But I am bald, and hardly ever walk
> by day, I'm the invalid of these rooms,
> stirring soups, awake in the half dark,
> not answering the phone when it rings.
>
> I never thought that life could get this small,
> that I would care so much about a cup,
> the taste of tea, the texture of a shawl,
> and whether or not I should get up.
>
> I'm not unhappy. I have learned to drift
> and sip. The smallest things are gifts.[4]

These two pieces of writing starkly illustrate the different focus and perspective of medical research and the patient. I present these accounts not to criticise the objectivity of the former, but to suggest the almost impossible task of moderating or coalescing the perspectives of each into an exchange between doctor and patient that can take seriously the needs of the patient and the concerns of clinical medicine and evidence-based practice. The extract from the *NEJM* reflects those concerns. What doctors need to know is what are the expected side effects, what proportion of patients do they affect, how potentially serious are they for the patient and whether they can be resolved – with time or additional treatment. Of course, the patient will be keenly interested in these issues, too, but for them, much more is at stake. For Darling, the effects of the treatment challenged her whole idea of herself: it was not in her plan to be 'bald at forty four'. She presents a rather charming (and we suspect tongue-in-cheek) picture of herself as a rather delicate middle-aged lady gracefully accepting the ageing process and fluttering a fan against menopausal hot flushes. Is this the 'age-matched' woman of the clinical trial? Darling suffers the side effect of 'fatigue', but in the poem we discover the consequence of this in her life. Her world has contracted. She ignores phone calls. She drifts about the house. She sleeps. She 'sips' (being too tired even to swallow or gulp) soups and tea.

When teaching medical students to be aware of the patient's perspective in their communication training, medical educators suggest that the medical students remember to ask about 'ideas, concerns and expectations', easily remembered by the acronym 'ICE'. Questions to the patient will uncover real concerns that can be answered and filled in by the doctor, such as how much time off work is involved, whether the treatment will hurt, what will happen next and the always lurking, 'Will I get better?' But what the doctor or medical student is unlikely to be asked is: 'How will I change?'; 'How will my idea of myself change?'; or, 'Will the feeling of "being me" change?' Patients can be left wondering, 'Who will the "me" without the breast/womb be?' or, later, 'Is that slow, sick, drowsy and confined person still me?' These existential and phenomenological consequences of treatment are often somewhat unexpected for the patient and usually not among the primary concerns of the clinician. Darling's poem, however, shows us how very real and pressing they are for the patient going through treatment and dealing with its consequences.

These questions are not just acute for the patient who is experiencing treatment but also for the relatives, friends and carers of the patient who are part of his world and who help define his view of his embodied self. Close relatives and friends will be affected by the patient's altered sense of himself within an episode of treatment: his relative or friend may seem distant, the patient feeling more comfortable within the world of the clinic than the domestic world that they have shared together. For doctors and other caregivers, involvement in the acts of treatment, especially if that treatment involves practical skills and their execution, may have profound implications for the ways in which they define themselves.

TREATMENT AND THE PATIENT

Turning first to the patient. Our story of Liz's treatment for her cervical pre-cancer illustrates the mismatch in experience and perspective between doctor and patient during the event. The routine and habit of the clinical staff is in stark contrast to the strangeness of the episode for the patient. Explanations are provided for the mechanics of the procedure but no thought is given to the possible flavour of the sensory experience for the patient. Pain is considered but not the 'sense of heat, the smell of burning flesh' that Liz finds so distressing. Strangeness piles upon strangeness as she has unexplained attachments slapped to her thigh, as she is scrutinised through the colposcope, which seems to threaten her 'exposed' rear end, and as she is touched by unseen instruments. Is it any wonder that Liz faints?

The fainting is not just a physical reaction to the procedure, but an existential response to the sudden reversal of her sense of being at home in her body. In handling, touching, manipulating and removing bits of the patient's body during the course of a treatment episode, the doctor is introducing a barrier of strangeness between the patient and that familiar flesh that has been her own (often unacknowledged) self for her conscious life. Jean Paul Sartre in *Being and Nothingness* explains this sense of alienation from the body:

> But as soon as we *know* the body- *i.e.*, as soon as we apprehend it in a purely cognitive intuition – we constitute it by that very intuition with the Other's knowledge (i.e., as it would never be for us by itself).[5]

During her treatment episode, Liz's body has become the object of a series of technical manipulations that are entirely unfamiliar to her. She can be 'earthed' in order for the diathermy to work. Her flesh is cut away while she is still awake and she can smell it burning. She is even invited to view on a screen a bit of herself that no woman would normally visually be able to confront. This is a real challenge to her sense of herself – her 'me' – and leaves her confused, scared and at a loss to recover and express what it is that she has lost, perhaps just for the time of the treatment, perhaps for even longer. Her treatment has forced her to think about her body through the concepts and language of medicine: through the point of view of 'the other' and 'as if [she] were the Other in relation to it'.[6]

This alienation from the body and fear of the unknown self is a common factor in patient accounts of severe illness. The journalist Melanie Reid, a keen sportswoman, suffered a spinal injury in a fall from her horse and lost the use of her legs. She continued to write her column for *The Times Magazine* throughout the period immediately after her injury and during her treatment. She suffers the same kind of physical reaction as Liz when forced to confront the bit of her that no longer felt like 'me':

> The first time my bed-head was raised high enough for me to catch sight of my legs, I felt physically sick. They looked like the Guy Fawkes [mannequins] we made as children for Bonfire Night, newspaper stuffed into old socks, ankles bent at unreal angles into discarded, puffy plimsolls. They weren't my legs at all; they were horrific, alien objects. The only way to describe the impact is to say I felt like I had suffered a compound fracture of the soul.[7]

This sense of alienation from parts of herself continues even during the treatment period. While she receives physiotherapy she begins to experience some sensation in her limbs but this is described in mechanical, rather than fleshly, terms: The nerves buzz away like a 'lawnmower' revving up for the first cut after winter, or like 'a computer attempting to reboot itself'.

Of course, the situation described by Reid and the treatment episode that Liz goes through are very different with respect to the demands they make on the patient's sense of self. Liz can walk away despite the trauma of her treatment experience and need not confront this alternative view of her body day by day, although some niggling remaining alienation and fear may remain. Reid does not have this choice. Her only option is to adapt.

The acclaimed historian Tony Judt has written recently of his experience of adaptation to motor neurone disease. There is no curative treatment for this problem; his treatment is care and company. However, when night falls he is left alone.

> During the day I can at least request a scratch, an adjustment, a drink, or simply a gratuitous replacement of my limbs – since enforced stillness for hours on end is not only physically uncomfortable but psychologically close to intolerable. ... But then comes the night.[8]

In the daytime Judt is occupied with interactions with carers and family members and – connected to this – with the treatment and care of his immobile body: the alternate placing of limbs to avoid pressure sores, the suctioning of phlegm from his throat in order to prevent aspiration, for example. However, at night he is left frustratingly and painfully unable to respond to the many physical signals that his body constantly throws up. In order to overcome the mental pain of this situation and the knowledge of his incurable condition, he retreats into his mind and his memory. His solution is to write in his head through the night and by this process of intensely focused thought become distracted from his physical state. Significantly, the technique he uses to capture the content and flow of the piece he is writing is to envisage his imagined active body moving around a chalet, packaging each thought in a separate cupboard or drawer in different rooms in sequence. He calls these 'memory chalets'.[9] When he comes to wake in the morning, he can re-enter the rooms he has pictured and moved around in his imagination, pull the memories from their hiding places and put them back together by dictating to his assistant.

As he describes it, this adaptation to his illness has two advantages. First, he is enabled to not feel constantly like a 'vegetable', which is how he often sees his physical self in the context of the total dependency he has on carers and those who treat the consequences of his illness: 'The minute I get an itch under my arm I become the vegetable again.'[10] As he can live a life of the mind, he still exists as himself in that domain; had he been a plumber, he suggests, the illness would have been a 'catastrophe'. The second advantage of his adaptation is a sense of control. He quotes the first line of a poem by Emily Dickinson: 'After great pain, a formal feeling comes.' His pain is psychological rather than physical, and the 'formal feeling' is one that he identifies as a sense of control over this devastating illness that allows him little leeway to be himself. The adaptation here is an attempt to recover the sense of me-ness that the illness has removed. It cannot be complete for Judt, as his physical self is 'vegetative', but his mind is active and he can roam free in his imagination.

Judt's case is an extreme one. He is unable to adapt in a way to recover himself fully physically and psychologically, but through an extreme effort of will and imagination, he can regain himself in his mind. This is a form of self-treatment – a way of adapting to altered circumstances that enables life to continue in a tolerable way. Treatment often includes the need to accept a differently functioning body: the need to interrupt a walk to take an inhaler in asthma, the use of a stick to improve walking after a knee replacement, or even the addition of glasses to improve poor vision. At first these tools become interruptions to what the patient may regard as 'normal' functioning, but if they are permanent additions to the patient's daily life, adaptation occurs. As Merleau-Ponty suggests, in allowing the body to function as near as possible to what was 'normal' before, over time these tools become part of the self and can lead eventually to a feeling of incompleteness when the tool is absent.[11] Spectacle wearers often remark that they feel naked without their glasses.

Adaptation to changed physical circumstances and body sense brought about by treatment is important for our ability to get through a treatment episode. The philosopher Havi Carel, in her moving account of her own serious illness, discusses the need to keep living well despite constant reminders of deteriorating physical functioning, such as the need to use oxygen while taking a short walk. She notes Martin Heidegger's characterisation of human existence as 'being able to be'.[12] Heidegger says that we think of our lives as meaningful because of the potential to do what we want and to become what we have the potential to be. Illness and its treatment bring human beings into contact with what Carel terms an 'inability to be'. Even self-limiting illnesses like influenza are a powerful reminder of how we have to withdraw from normal activities for a while to recover or while treatment takes its course. For a time the patient has to come to terms with the fact that an 'inability to be' has to become for them a way of being. Patients undergoing intensive care are the most dramatic examples of 'not being'. They may be unconscious and totally dependent on others for all physical functions. But even Liz during the course of her LLETZ treatment had to face realities about her body that affected her sense of being and not being herself. As Carel argues, our need to continue to exist and to manage daily life in the face of illness and its treatment and the altered sense of being that these bring require adaptation and acceptance of inability. Reid in her response to the early stages of recovery from spinal injury is still suffering acutely from inability to be, but Judt, through an effort of imagination and acute self-knowledge, has discovered a new way to be. As Carel concludes:

> Acknowledging an inability and learning to see it as part of life's terrain are important lessons that illness can teach at any age. This knowledge enables the ill person to embrace the unable self as part and parcel of human existence. By having a more balanced view of life as combining ability and inability, illness can become more accepted and less disruptive. In addition, the ability to

> accept an unable self can be the first step towards answering a pressing question for all ill people: given that I am ill, can I still have a good life?[13]

The subject of adaptation to the outcomes of illness and the changes in being and ability that are brought with illness are the subjects of the final book of this series, and these ideas will be pursued in more detail there. But, as I have suggested above, an episode of treatment may for the first time in an illness starkly bring patients into a realisation of their bodily existence in a way that changes them and brings about the need to adapt and reconsider their own sense of being. Despite the alienation from the body that the experience of illness and its treatment can bring it is possible to adapt and reach a new sense of one-ness with the body in its altered state. Treatment offered – and the role of the physician in the way that that treatment is delivered – can either assist or get in the way of that adaptation. I will consider this in the final section of this chapter. But alongside the patient, it is important to consider the perspectives of those who are closest to him in his daily life and what a treatment episode may mean for them as they support the patient or just watch and wait.

TREATMENT AND CLOSE OTHERS

Relatives, especially partners and spouses, may feel fractured in their relationship with their partner during the course of a treatment episode. There may be an exclusive focus by the patient on his illness and on getting through the treatment that may lead to the development of intense (at least on the patient's side) relationships with carers and clinicians that exclude partners. In Volume 2 of this series we discussed the idea of 'intimacy' within the clinical encounter and noted the characteristics of clinical interactions that make this possible. Examinations involve physical touch, sometimes of a very intimate nature, and doctors need to ask questions that may delve more deeply into a patient's concerns than his closest friends and relatives feel able to. Once a treatment episode is initiated by the clinician, the patient's dependence becomes greater while in some ways the intense interest of the doctor becomes less. The difficult business of diagnosis is now complete (unless it needs to be reconsidered) and now treatment protocols need to be followed. For patients, it is different. Treatment is the crucial stage of the interaction with their clinicians, as so much depends on whether it goes well or not and on the eventual outcome. As with Rachel's dependence on Dax, her diabetic treatment nurse in our story, it can seem that only the doctor or nurse understands what the patient is going through or what she needs during a period of treatment.

There are also potentially more fundamental effects on relationships that are not to do with shifts in allegiance. I have already discussed the possible effect of treatment on the patient's sense of themselves, and that alteration can affect others, too. The operative removal of some part of the body that is, for example, defining of a woman's sexuality – most obviously breasts or even womb and ovaries – can affect the patient's ability to feel sexual or even to feel like a 'real woman'. Such disruptions to a patient's bodily identity may lead to distancing from those that they are closest to, at least until adaptation to the change is achieved.

As the writer Hilary Mantel describes in her account of her husband's admission to hospital for an emergency operation, distancing is most acute when the patient is removed from home for treatment elsewhere. She describes a terrible day waiting for the outcome of her husband's operation:

> One of my brothers sits with me while I wait at home for news; I don't go to the hospital because it is vast and once there I cannot be sure to be in the right part of it to get the news and yesterday's experience teaches me that I would be deeply unwelcome. By mid-afternoon no one has called me. I begin to suspect he has got so far he may never come back. When I phone the unit that claims to expect him, they can tell me nothing. Must still be in theatre, they say; but it's clear they don't care, it isn't their responsibility. Have they just mislaid him? That seems possible. They take my number and say they will tell me if he turns up. By this time I don't believe a word of it. Five o'clock, an irritable man tells me off: 'When you phone you take us away from our patients.' ... This is the worst day of my life.[14]

When eventually she gets to see her husband in intensive care, the gap between them has widened still further, accentuated by the physical surroundings and the intensity of the experience she has had that has not been shared by her husband.

> In here [the intensive care unit] there is neither day nor night, but a reverent hush, a reassuring bleeping and hissing of machines. The patient is awake and cracking jokes. We gape down at him, out of breath. We do not tell him, at this stage, about the hours we have passed, their strange texture, how gradually the drip of dismay entered our veins, then fear and desolation.

Mantel's account is full of the horror of realising that illness and treatment have the power very suddenly to disrupt the closest ties that have developed between people over years, and to make people, perhaps only temporarily, strangers to each other. In our stories of Jen and Geoff, Jen is horrified by the idea that her husband, in his demented state, may not even notice the changes that her illness and its treatment have brought about – even to the extent of him being unaware of her 'non-being' in death.

Some close partners may have the opposite experience if their loved one is suffering pain or unpleasant symptoms. They may actually experience some of the physical symptoms that their partner is suffering. One well-recognised example of this is Couvade Syndrome, when expectant fathers suffer from symptoms related to pregnancy and even experience abdominal pains while their partners are in labour. There are many, less dramatic, examples of this phenomenon. Hilary Mantel in the diary account I quoted from above noted that while waiting in hospital with her husband before his operation, 'our breathing seemed to synchronise', such was the physical empathy between the two of them.[15] In Gwyneth Lewis's epic poem, *A Hospital Odyssey*, Maris does battle for her husband against his illness in the corridors and wards of her fictional hospital and finds herself hospitalised as well:

> 'Hold on!' cried Maris, 'it's my husband who is ill,
> not me.' 'N-n-n-nonsense,' Matron stuttered.
> 'He's poorly, you're married, you have a virtual
> disease and, therefore, you have to be cured
> of your neuroses. The treatment is hard
>
> but utterly worth it.' 'I must confess,
> my body's partnered to his, I do feel sick
> if he's laid up.' Obediently, Maris undressed,
> pulled on a hospital gown – you know, that classic
> backless blue the opposite of chic –
>
> and climbed into bed.[16]

Maris feels that her body is 'partnered' to her husband's and thus that she also needs treatment when he is ill. Whether this experience is metaphorical, a physical reality or expressive of a desire to cleave to one's partner when they are in distress and to fend off the dislocating effects of illness and treatment on a close relationship, its existence should remind doctors, nurses and others of the importance of caring both for patients and their relatives during a treatment episode.

TREATMENT AND THE DOCTOR

What I have said in the foregoing sections suggests that doctors, in their role as initiators, participants and overseers in treatment episodes, have the capacity to affect the experience of treatment for patients and those close to them in ways that lie outside of the doctor's medical prescribing skills or surgical dexterity and anatomical understanding. It is important not to overburden clinicians with tasks and perspectives that would interfere with the imperative to deliver evidence-based treatment, but for those treatments to be effective, it is important for doctors to consider how they 'treat of' the patient, in the sense I explored at the beginning of this chapter.

As an episode of treatment advances, the doctor's idea of the patient – how they 'treat of' the patient – may undergo a change. As we discussed in the first volume of this series, *Symptom*, patients arrive at the GP surgery with symptoms that are un-sorted. In the mind of the consulting doctor, therefore, the patient has no disease category and can only be viewed as a person with a set of symptoms and signs. As that problem becomes clearer – the illness is named and the doctor decides on the most effective treatment – the nature of the interaction and its outcome develops an inevitable likely course and the doctor's way of thinking and the kind of language she uses to speak to the patient begins to take on patterns familiar to the doctor but alien to the patient – or at least alien until time allows adaptation to a new sense of understanding for the patient of his own body.

Returning to the account that Sartre gives of this issue, which I discussed briefly in the first section of this chapter, he reveals the problems that are inevitable in interactions between people (doctor and patient) whose understandings of the body, the impact of illness and its treatment are so disparate:

> In order that any knowledge which the Other [i.e. doctor in the present context] has of my body and which he communicates to me by language may give to my body-for-me a structure of a particular type, it is necessary that this knowledge be applied to an object and that my body already be an object for me.[17]

The implication here is that the first step that the patient has to take in beginning to understand what illness and treatment mean for his sense of being is to objectify his body – to see it and think about it from a perspective outside of himself, and that perspective is supplied – at least at first – by the doctor. Sartre goes on:

> The illness which I suffer can aim at its In-itself; that is precisely in its being-for-others. At this moment I *know* it; that is I aim at it in its dimension of being which escapes me, at the face of which it turns towards Others, and my aim is impregnated with the wisdom which language has brought to me; – *i.e.*, I utilize instrumental concepts which come to me from the Other, and which I should in no case have been able to form by myself or think of directing upon my body. It is by means of the Other's concepts that I *know* my body.

More will be said later in this volume about object–subject relationships (*see* Chapter 3). What I have argued in this chapter is that the experience of one's body through illness can be alienating – or it can reveal a 'dimension of being which escapes [us]', as Sartre would have it. Often this alienation is most acutely revealed (as in the story of Liz) in a treatment episode where we must face the reality of how our own familiar flesh is seen, named, handled and sensed (in Liz's case, smelled) by others. Doctors are the 'Other' who confront patients first with ideas of their bodies as objects in this way, through the language that they use and ways in which they may handle the patient physically during treatment. Being aware of the potential strangeness of this new body and being sensitive to the patient's need for time to allow adaptation to a new sense of themselves is important in order for treatment to be successful. Havi Carel wisely suggests some questions that a doctor can ask of her patients:

> [H]ow has illness or disability changed your life? What aspects of it affect you the most? How can those effects be made up for? These kinds of phenomenologically informed questions open a space for the creative adaptivity that can enable a good life even with illness.[18]

Finally, having considered the effects of a treatment episode on a patient's body sense, it is important also to note that the treatment of patients can have implications for doctors and their own relationships with their bodies. We have already discussed the intimacy of the relationship between doctor and patient, which is mediated by the need for doctors to use their clinical skills of examination (*see* Volume 2, Chapter 7). In that chapter we quoted a passage from Kathleen Jamie's work that described a cool, clinical relationship between doctor and patient but revealed a deep understanding by the doctor of the diseased physical body that was revealed by her expert use of a clinical tool:

> Leaning across the bed behind him, the doctor placed her stethoscope at precise points on Phil's back, and began to listen. As she listened, she created around herself a screen of privacy. Her eyes disengaged. She folded herself into the stethoscope, in toward Phil's back, attending to the sound as a musician might. Then she began concentrating on an area midway down his right side. She was tracking something within his body, moving the stethoscope an inch to the left, and inch to the right then back again, as if comparing two notes. Suddenly she was satisfied, and leaned back, tugging the stethoscope out of her ears.[19]

I am revisiting this passage because it illustrates very strikingly the absolute focus the doctor gives to the exploration of the sound through the contact of the stethoscope. It is the kind of focus we may observe from a concert pianist 'losing himself' in the creative act. There is no consciousness of the piano, as of the instrument through which the doctor is 'tracking' the sound: attention is complete. And the conclusion is accurate diagnosis and appropriate treatment. The key points are that the mind is focused on an intention: that of detecting the pathognomonic sound that tells you that this is pneumonia, and the instrument is a means, in expert hands, to achieve that end.

This unawareness of the instrument of examination or treatment is a feature of habit and expertise, and not something experienced by the beginner. As doctors in training or apprenticed surgeons learn to use the tools of their trade (including stethoscope and tendon hammer or, more sophisticatedly, laparoscope or biopsy loop) the self-conscious awareness of these instruments in their hands begins to dissolve. As the surgeon gains increasing expertise in operating she becomes less able to distinguish between her body and the instrument she is manipulating.

Matthew Ratcliffe describes this phenomenon as one of 'extended touch', where it becomes unclear to the operator where his body ends and the inert instrument begins.[20] Experienced clinicians will comment on the consistency of an organ examined by them at a distance: It is 'craggy' or 'rubbery', and when cut during surgery or biopsy, it may be 'gritty' or 'smooth'. In some way, it seems, these consistencies are 'felt' by the examiner in his hand. They are in fact 'felt' by the end of the instrument or the teeth of the biopsy forceps, but the hand/mind of the clinician fuse in the act of sorting out the diagnosis or carrying out treatment. It takes time for clinicians to become habituated to the use of instrumentation. Practise is essential for adaptation of this sort to occur and surgeons in training will often go about their rounds continually tying and retying one-handed knots so that their fingers begin to automatically make the movements. Ian McEwan captures the manual skill of his expert neurosurgeon, Guy Perowne, at work in his novel *Saturday*:

> While Sally closed up a patient Perowne went next door to relieve an elderly lady of her trigeminal neuralgia, her tic douloureux. These minor operations can still give him pleasure – he likes to be fast and accurate. He slipped a gloved forefinger into the back of her mouth to feel the route, then, with barely a glance at the image intensifier, slid a long needle through the inside of her cheek, all the way up to the trigeminal ganglion.[21]

The slightest slip in this kind of procedure could have ghastly consequences for the patient, but Perowne's confidence as a result of the fusion between his body and the instruments he is using is such that he barely needs to look at what he is doing – it is all done by touch.

Thus the body sense of the treating clinician changes as she develops her expertise in operating or in other practical treatment delivery. This change becomes part of her identity as a person.

In summary then, treatment can have profound effects on patients' and doctors' own senses of themselves. For patients, these effects can be temporary or permanent, and if long lasting they can lead in turn to adaptation that enables patients to continue with their lives. The changes for doctors will last through their working lives as they continue to practise their expertise in treating patients. There may be consequences for doctors as individuals when they stop working and face not only loss of work but also loss of the body habits that have become part of their physical selves. Treatment episodes can affect relationships with close relatives and friends in ways not apparent to doctors or even to the patients themselves. Doctors, in their capacity as prescribers and deliverers of treatment, have an important role that goes beyond the physical or pharmacological exchanges of therapy to mediating the broader effects of those exchanges on patients' lives.

REFERENCES

1 Darling J. Chemotherapy. In: Darling, J. *Sudden Collapses in Public Places*. Todmorden, Lancashire: Arc Publications; 1993. p. 50.
2 Balint M. *The Doctor, His Patient and the Illness*. London: Churchill Livingston; 1957.
3 Shapiro CL *et al*. Side effects of adjuvant treatment of breast cancer. *NEJM*. 2001; **344**(26): 1997–2008.
4 Darling J, op. cit. p. 50.
5 Sartre J-P. *Being and Nothingness*. Oxon: Routledge; 2003 [1943]. p. 378. Emphasis in original.
6 Sartre J-P. *Being and Nothingness*. Oxon: Routledge; 2003 [1943]. p. 379.
7 Reid M. Spinal column. *The Times Magazine*. 5 June, 2010. p. 10.
8 Judt T. Night. *Guardian Review*. 16 January, 2010. p. 27.
9 Judt T. Interviewed on BBC Radio 4's *No Triumph, No Tragedy*. 29 June.
10 Judt T, ibid.
11 Merleau-Ponty M. *Phenomenology of Perception*. (Trans. C Smith). London: Routledge; 1962. p. 166.
12 Carel H. *Illness: the cry of the flesh*. Stocksfield: Acumen; 2008. p. 66.
13 Carel H, op. cit. p. 70.
14 Mantel H. Diary. *London Review of Books*. 2008; **30**: 40–1.
15 Mantel H, op. cit. p. 41.
16 Lewis G. *A Hospital Odyssey*. Highgreen, Northumberland: Bloodaxe Books; 2010. p. 24.
17 Sartre J-P, op. cit. p. 378.
18 Carel H, op. cit. p. 88.
19 Jamie K. *Findings*. London: Sort of Books; 2005. p. 103.
20 Ratcliffe M. *Feelings of Being*. Oxford: OUP; 2008. p. 91 (boundaries section).
21 McEwan I. *Saturday*. London: Jonathan Cape; 2005. p. 7.

2

Wonderful treatment

MARTYN EVANS

INTRODUCTION

A friend of mine once had the misfortune to suffer acute appendicitis and be admitted to hospital for emergency surgery. The operation was uneventful and wholly successful, my friend recovered in a manner and at a rate that was typical for his age (he was at the time in his forties) and he was discharged, went home, and soon resumed normal daily life. Notwithstanding the original misfortune, the whole episode was otherwise entirely unremarkable from a medical viewpoint. However, telling me about it later, my friend described the familiar signs and symptoms of his digestive system starting to work again as he convalesced and, as he put it, from his perspective as a biologist, 'It was wonderful to observe my digestive system – my body – coming back to life.'

The treatment involved, in his case appendicectomy, is in biophysical terms well understood, as is why it should be needed and how it works. It is, from a surgical perspective, entirely ordinary and routine, even mechanical – hardly the stuff of wonder. And yet, as my friend – himself a trained biological scientist – observed, its result *was* in part wonderful. In this chapter I want to explore, and defend, that remark, and I want to do so in the context not merely of my friend's treatment but of the idea of treatment as such. Successful or otherwise, all treatments, I will suggest, are at least partly wonderful.

This is perhaps such a surprising claim that it needs some clarification here, right at the outset. Three of our patients might protest against the claim – Jake hotly; Liz and, perhaps, Jen in more muted and inward terms. Jake's defiant "I don't want any more tubes stuck up and through me. I'm not a freak... I don't want any more of those bloody tests and I don't want any bloody pills either" is no endorsement of the wonder of treatment. Liz's treatment elicits her twitches, groans, revulsion, nausea – as well as her disbelief that any woman might actually want to watch the proceedings on a television monitor. Jen endures humiliation at 'her body letting her down'; 'How many times do I have to do this? How will I ever cope?' She is amazed at what she does cope with; but any wonder here seems directed at her own resilient spirit rather than at medicine's efforts.

So let my clarification start with what I am *not* claiming – that individual treatments are unfailingly occasions for grateful joy. Even when they are free of discomfort, easily tolerated and rapidly effective I am not claiming that, in showing this, we have disclosed what makes them wonderful. Nor is their wonder a matter of technical bravura. Admittedly, it might be said that, in the accumulated observations that led to a treatment's being conjectured and refined, or in the intelligence through which theoretical understandings of the body explain how a treatment can work, or in the meticulous practicalities of the way that a treatment is administered, all treatments (or at least all those that work well) represent wonderful gains in our understanding and therapeutic capacity. But such wonderfulness is temporary, simply part of our acknowledgement of something novel, our relieved greeting of another victory in a long struggle. The *enduring* wonderfulness of treatment lies elsewhere, and indeed it permeates the very idea of treatment.

Treatment consists – and its wonderfulness is provoked – in the interaction between the therapeutic procedure and the person treated: in the inducing of change in the bodily make-up of the patient; in the deliberate constructive alteration of the patient's embodied experience; in short, in *meddling in the flesh* of another person. What is wonderful is that this is possible; that it works as often as it does; and, most of all, that it works because our world and our experience of the world are embodied in our flesh.

To change our flesh is to change – hopefully, for the better – the way that we experience the world. This embodiment, of which we are forcibly reminded every time we try to affect it by direct physical intervention, is enduringly wonderful. From embodiment's wonderfulness, the wonderfulness of treatment directly stems.

BODILY WONDER

Ordinary living, being and doing: what we take for granted

I have noticed elsewhere[1] the virtues of Rene Leriche's remark that 'health is life lived in the silence of the organs'.[2] Shrewd though it be, the remark has its shortcomings, among them that it ignores the obvious fact that the skin is one organ whose silence is not a precondition for health. In all sorts of ordinary doings and undertakings in daily life our skin will register all sorts of sensations, including discomforts and irritations. When we try to stop still for a moment our attention is sometimes freed to register these discomforts. It happens that I am writing the present lines on a laptop computer which for once does indeed sit in my lap; I'm virtually encased in an old armchair, perched just in front of the full-height windows of an upper-floor lounge, looking out over the garden. Right now I would describe myself as perfectly healthy, although – now that I pause to register the facts – my arms are irritated by the rough wool of my sweater, the cushion in the small of my back seems always in the wrong place, my chair forces upon me a maddeningly crooked posture, I've an excessively acidic tang in my mouth from drinking strong tea earlier and my stomach is restless for some food; and, finally, my reading glasses make the garden through the window seem a dim and misty place. None of these discomforts seems to have any bearing on my conviction that I am in normal health; each of them, however, is a reminder of the essential physicality of experience, whether as foreground or as background.

Our bodies make our worlds just as, in turn, they are made by those worlds.[(i)] When I was younger I liked the appearance of my hands – small, neat, lithe, a pianist's hands as well as a furniture-maker's hands. Now (thanks partly to years of exposure to the sawdust and solvents of the furniture trade) my hands look considerably older than I do, and I will consider this change further in a little while. But, despite their appearance, my hands continue to work, and well enough. They act in the world, and yet I have not the faintest conception of how my thoughts and intentions, in terms of the words that I want to type, can possibly actuate the accomplishments of my hands, in terms of sequences of keystrokes correctly delivered; more generally, I have not – and it seems to me that I cannot have – any true and deep conception of how my will is manifest in physical action. (The best account – that of the German philosopher Schopenhauer, according to whom the action is nothing other than the intention observed from outside, and the intention nothing other than the action experienced from the inside – solves the puzzle only by attempting to *dis*solve it, almost to deny it as a puzzle at all.[4]) Equally, experience is the inward expression of outward events and processes: yet I have not the slightest conception – and it seems to me that I cannot have – of how the physical, material sequences of touch and sensation and perception become manifest in the non-material reality of felt, qualitative experience.

This brings into sharp focus the primary ground of treatment's wonderfulness – the incredible constitution of experience, even the possibility of experience, by that subtly and minutely organised substance that we call flesh. Nowhere

(i) In this and the subsequent two paragraphs I use the words in which I present these thoughts in discussion of the corresponding points in a paper on wonder in the clinical context.[3]

is this more graphically laid bare for us than by the sometimes-questionable products of Gunter von Hagens's 'plastinated' anatomical dissections. Even before we come to the dazzling array of neural circuitry within which we take consciousness to have its chief administration, the possibility of continued animal life lies spectacularly in the visceral manifold lying with the chest and abdomen. These engines of circulation, respiration and digestion cleave together in a complex, coloured and congested heap of flesh; its untidy, haphazard scrambling nonetheless conforms closely to a regular blueprint – a blueprint that sustains all higher forms of air-breathing, warm-blooded, locomotive life.

This gaudy pile, in equal measure revolting and wondrous to behold, is our inner permit to exist at all; without it, our brains and sensory organs can neither function nor arise in the first place. It is the 'soft machinery'[5] that causes Liz's world briefly to swim and dim as the shocking aspects of her treatment fully register, and that turns Jen's bed abruptly into a latrine; yet upon this machinery they – we – depend utterly and moment-by-moment. It is the boiler-room of fleshly life; and our life is a fleshly one.[6]

The dazzling richness of perceptual experience

Nowhere perhaps is the 'taken-for-grantedness' of our condition more remarkable than in ordinary perceptual experience. We accept without question just those five primary senses through which we engage with the world, even construct it, and we give barely a thought to the other ways in which the world might – must – appear to other kinds of creatures: we take the world at face value, presuming that the face it shows to us is of necessity its real face. Just as effortlessly we embrace the contrasting modalities of the different individual senses, and their fusion in a single, continuous world of multi-modal experience. Thus we accept without question the activeness of touch, and we have no difficulty intermingling active tactile experience with the helpless passivity of hearing. We accept without question the precise and stable structural repertoire of the illuminated world within our incredibly finely-grained visual field, alongside the rich chaos of fleeting, evocative, often un-nameable swirls of scent and flavour that assail our senses of smell and taste: the velvet pink petals and heady scent of an opened damask rose offer a single, albeit complex, fused experience. And we almost invariably overlook proprioception – our inward, 'blindfolded' knowledge of our own moment-by-moment orientation, posture, extension – in whose absence we couldn't walk or raise a spoonful of food to our mouths without constant visual monitoring and correction of our movements.[7]

Each of our senses can give us pleasure, and each can give us disgust – although now it becomes more apparent that our reactions, be they of delight or revulsion, involve thinking and imagining directly in the identification of what it is we sense or perceive. We don't see or touch or hear things innocently:

they carry meaning for us even *before* actual sensation (which is in part what sensory *re*cognition comes to). Even smell and taste, which might seem to affect our experience with particularly unavoidable immediacy, can be modified by expectation and imagination (a smell like strong cheese is enjoyable if it is clearly associated with actual strong cheese, and anything but enjoyable if its source lies elsewhere, and this remains true even if the source is a matter of what we merely believe rather than actually know to be true). Sensory experience can be frustratingly 'thin' – think of the use of sensory deprivation as a punishment – or it can be overwhelmingly intense, even in the absence of direct stimulation of pain. Sights and sounds and flavours can be simply too much to take in all at once; we have limiting comfortable levels of sensory experience, as well as enjoyable or aversive characteristic objects of that experience.

Any and all of this might have been otherwise, but it is not otherwise; the facts of our perceptual life are as they are. Our sensory experience is contingent, intense, close-knit, almost entirely continuous, and rich beyond measure. At the same time it is curiously limited: we have no intrinsic sensory experience of mass; we cannot feel magnetism; we are blind to all but a fraction of radiated energy frequencies; we have only a coarse awareness of pressure variation; we cannot 'meter' the passing of time; and so on. Perhaps above all, though, our sensory experience is unconsciously *integrated*: we have no awareness of the joining together of the multiple worlds of sound, space, sight and smell into a single world of embodied existence. They are co-fabricated in our brains, fused with our equally-unquestioning sense of our own identity and continuity, into what Kant intriguingly called the 'manifold of perception'.[8] The world's muted daily ordinariness – but also its breathtaking dynamism and beauty – arise in and through this glorious symphony of sensory embodiment.

And its greatest glory is also its greatest wonder – the wonder that we can have this inward, *felt* quality of sensation at all: the wonder that sensory experience is not simply *information* enabling us to negotiate a survival in the world around us but rather the vivid aliveness of being embodied creatures in a material world. Our experience *is* the world – a world of externalities that, in and through our consciousness (and presumably the consciousness of many, many forms of animal life), has been given a qualitative, felt, 'inside'. Nothing, it seems to me, is more wonderful than this. Only slightly less wonderful is its modulation by medicine.

The material grounding of behaviour, in sickness and health

Not only do we sense and experience the world around us: we act in and on it. And just as our perception is the experiential 'interior' of material things and processes, so our actions are the experiential 'interior' of the processes by which we govern and are governed by the material world. We habitually and unhesitatingly act and move fluently; we think, do, respond to and immerse ourselves in a rich, multi-sensory and above all embodied world – doing all of this generally without conscious effort; fluidly, often carelessly; mostly without wonder.

Our baseline for effort or conscious attention rests both upon unthinking embodied fluency and upon the automatic coherence that we somehow make of our kaleidoscopic sensory experience. Equally, it seems that our baseline for intentional action is blindly shaped by patterned physical interactions at the biochemical and biomechanical levels. We are almost never aware of these interactions, some of them in turn governed by unalterable patterns in our genes and others by adaptive patterns in our nervous systems. We can do nothing about (though perhaps we could do little without) the instincts that are characteristic of our biological species, and that fit us generally to survive in physical terms. Our 'primitive reactions'[9] are our broadly-shared genetic blueprint coming to life, for the most part protectively, in our outward behaviour – turning abruptly at a sound or at a tap on the shoulder, recoiling from painful or disgusting stimuli, scratching an itch, seeking out warmth and light and comfort, enjoying sounds within a certain range of pitch and volume and consonance, trembling when afraid, hesitating at the unknown, acknowledging the human face and its likenesses, attending to the sound of human (and other mammalian) infants, and – I dare say – sometimes gazing in rapt wonder at what is remote.

These reactions are built into us regardless of when or where we are born. Other reactions come about, or are at least activated, by the cultural and social environment surrounding us. Our social habits, our learned conformities, become automatic and in time quite as unconscious (subjectively speaking) as our biological reactions. This is true also of our idiosyncratic behaviour, our individual habits that had perhaps a conscious beginning but develop a life and compulsion of their own, moulding the way we speak, act and think.

The first wonderful thing about all of this – comparable to the wonder of materially grounded perceptual experience – is how essentially simple chemical interactions can, in predictable combination, generate reliable, repeated, complex behaviour. This is already wonderful enough in the case of more specialised creatures than ourselves: for what essentially chemical combination of the actions of genes could possibly 'code' in a reliable, causal, manner for the building of a bird's nest, still less for a social artefact such as a beehive, where the interactions of different individuals and their roles make a kind of unconscious joint authorship of such beautiful structures? But, staggeringly, in our own case the mechanical influences of our genetic complement enable enormous flexibility and adaptability; they produce our seemingly unopposable mixture of curiosity, risk-taking, individual aggrandisement and collective prudence.

The second wonderful thing about embodied action is what it *feels* like, in ordinary health. We take for granted (to the point of almost never finding time to recognise and revel in its wonderfulness) our fluent, carefree, agency in the world. Our experience of our actions is of a physical body moved by will; yet our material reality is of a will both fuelled and constrained by physicality. We feel as though our bodies enact our will; it would be truer to say that our wills express our bodies. The Cartesian conceit under which we normally labour would be wonderful enough, of course; however, no less wonderful is this idea of channelling, into concrete deliberate action in the world around us, new combinations of those felt impulses and possibilities that are fabricated in our flesh by genes, instincts and habits.

To be in ordinary health *is*, in part, to be and to act in this ordinary way, taking our ordinary being and our ordinary acting for granted, utterly unaware of what underlies them.

Illness and other metamorphoses

Perhaps this taken-for-grantedness explains our sense of absurd contingency about falling ill, a sense positioned somewhere amid bafflement, outrage and embarrassment. One moment we are engaged in the ordinary affairs of living – absorbed, preoccupied or bored as the case may be – and the next moment all of our calculations are set aside and all our taken-for-grantedness is thrust back in our teeth. Like accidents, illnesses should not happen, but they do. They should happen to other people, in other lives, yet they happen to us, in ours. They should not happen now, so inconveniently, but in the future when we can afford the luxury of the time and attention that illnesses demand; but they will not wait for us. Or they impertinently remind us of our own behavioural choices, the risks to which we've exposed our health; and it seems to us (as John Diamond brutally illustrates in his autobiographical *C: Because cowards get cancer too ...*[10]) that we were unfairly dealt with when we fail to 'get away' with risks run blithely and successfully by others.

However, in bringing about unwelcome change, illnesses serve doubly to emphasise the general point that concerns me here: they remind us forcibly of the materiality of our existence, and they remind us of how tightly we are bound to it. Perhaps it takes as much self-mastery to be able to ignore pleasures as to be able to ignore pains, but illnesses change not only how we can be (our moment-to-moment experience) but what we can do and attempt. Moral fortitude may help us bear up under immobility and weakness, but it can do little about the basic limitations that these force upon us. The disruption and alteration of our ordinary existence and function is in its way only one more manifestation of the wonder of embodied experience. While it lasts, illness transforms the world – something as worthy of wonder as it is, for a time, shocking – but it also, astonishingly, can transform our own materiality.

Of course, whether well or ill, we are all helpless passengers in the long, slow, train-crash that is ageing. The poet Philip Larkin compared the hands of the elderly to toads – pudgy, wrinkled, inflexible and mottled.[11] Two 'toads', unhappily, now squat on the keyboard of my laptop; they are part of me, and my access to the world through them is the same as it ever was; but falling within my own view they strike me unfavourably, as (I imagine) they do others. Blooms that are now rather shrivelled, they are still my trusted ambassadors in the world immediately around me, but they no longer advertise or introduce my former, youthful self. Yet – occupational injuries and spills apart – I have not consciously brought about this metamorphosis. I have not even tried to stop its effects with moisturising or alleged 'anti-ageing' creams, as so many people, men included these days, try to do. My hands' metamorphosis is part of me yet independent of me. And it forcibly reminds me of the contingency of my body. Here it is – a bag of meat and offal and bones, as Bryan Magee brutally puts it[12] – that has slowly, over a lifetime, extruded itself out of available matter and space to occupy one (and one only) of infinitely many possible variations on the basic human form. I'm stuck with it; I'm stuck *as* it. Here my toad hands squat in front of me and neither I nor they can do a thing about it in any fundamental sense.

But although all of this sounds rather sour and resentful, it is also recognition of something wonderful. Toad-like or not, my over-aged hands are one illustrative aspect of the wonder of the gross morphological changes the human body undergoes over a lifetime. A typical human proceeds from conception through explosive gestation and live birth, to a parade of changing body forms and facial appearances in infancy, childhood, puberty, maturity, reproductive prime, the long middle years, elderly decline, death and disintegration: every aspect of this deserves wonder.

I recently gazed, transfixed, at the youngest occupant of an American paediatric intensive care unit. Not only had I no *personal* connection with this desperately fragile infant; more shockingly, given the child's heartbreaking prematurity, his appearance was such that at one level it was hard to recognise between us any *classificatory* connection as humans either. The tiniest living human I have ever seen with my own eyes, this looked more like a shrunken rubber balloon with spider limbs and a perishable, convulsing, cling-film surface. Intubated, bandaged, blindfolded, wrenched by natural mishap from the uterus where he might have flourished, clinging to life by means that were as much metaphysical as physical (I mean, his sheer will-to-live), he had become the pulsing junction-box for all of the sterile electro-mechanical machinery around and partly within him. In safer circumstances it is obvious that through this crucible-stage we have all, each one of us, voyaged – foetally curled and amniotically swathed rather than spreadeagled supine upon a cotton sheet in sterile air. This infant had wonder within him: against all odds he still lived (and, perhaps, lives still; an email enquiry would disclose the facts but I have not the courage to send it). Yet also he had wonder around him, in the institutional love – there is no other word – that invests such technical bravura in his struggle to live another day: and furthermore he emanated wonder in the invitation to see him as one of us.

It is remarkable that those who know us as individuals recognise a continuing underlying experiential unity – we might, though need not, call it 'identity' – through the gross outward changes (a favourite party game challenges participants to recognise their friends from childhood photographs); but in some ways it is still more remarkable that we recognise this continuity in our own experience: that a rich 'I' persists doggedly and, in later years, stoically, through physical metamorphosis of a kind that, if compressed, would be the stuff of nightmares.

In a sense, an intense compression of this sort actually *is* involved in the metamorphosis of illness. This can be acute and frightening, as Jane Macnaughton noted in the case of the child whose face 'disappeared' as her connective tissue desiccated (albeit temporarily) before her parents' horrified gaze.[13] But the metamorphosis is still remarkable even in less extreme cases: weight may be gained or lost in significant amounts; limbs and joints swell alarmingly with inflammation or oedema; there may be colour and complexion changes in fever; fluids may accumulate or leak out; there may be unorthodox growth – new tissues in new shapes, tumours, scars, keloids. Or there may be a 'kinetic' metamorphosis – a change in the nature and range of movement, a speeding up, a slowing down, spasms, rigidity, tremor. And so on. To us who – as we often believe in times of health – 'inhabit' our bodies, it becomes clear during illness that we *are* our bodies, for better or worse, and that our bodies are changing in a way that seems to be at odds with our continuity as selves.

Wondrously, of course, the metamorphoses of illness often go into reverse, sometimes just as quickly as they came about. We often do recover our former poise, posture, balance, watertight-ness, colour, odour, mass and shape (or at any rate most of it), with perhaps a residue of the change left in terms of scarring or stiffness as a longer-term legacy. Again, the continuity of the self persists through the metamorphosis. However, sometimes metamorphosis is not merely a result of a treatment; it is constituted by the treatment. This is typical of surgery – the cutting out and removal of obstructive or intrusive or dangerously broken flesh. For Liz the pervasive, persistent horror of her own treatment was the excision of a biopsy with an electrical loop: "...a sense of heat, the smell of burning flesh. This smell was the worst thing of all." Part of her had been both removed and, unavoidably, presented to her nostrils for what it had been changed into: burnt meat. This is a truly graphic form of what I earlier called 'meddling in the flesh'. For the physician, the experience is doubtless masked by routine; but, for Liz, a conscious patient, it is an existential threat, a reminder that what can in the right circumstances be appetising is also, in the wrong circumstances, a vignette of fiery death.

Those who administer such treatments do well to be mindful of their ambiguity, and this is equally true of far more mundane things than excision.

When Jen's cancer nurse brings her a wig in preparation for the impending loss of her hair, Jen is transported back to her youth and to the beauty of 'her swinging chestnut bob ... her best asset'. Perhaps her hair is no longer chestnut, and indeed its greying and crisping are part of Jen's life-cycle metamorphosis, but it still connects her with the selves she is losing – her own and Geoff's alike in their handsome youth, Geoff's now in most senses, given his withdrawn and unwitting state. The wig is kindly meant, a form of palliative treatment, but for the moment at least it is for Jen anything but a comfort.

When we do recover, it is of course a wonderful thing in every sense to regain ordinary embodiment and perception and function and self-experience. In terms of ordinary embodiment, when my friend coolly watched over his own recovery from appendicectomy, what was at stake for him as a biologist was, among other things, a kind of existential demonstration of the principles of biochemistry and physiology. That gaudy 'heap' of viscera had suffered the insult of surgery, ridden the blow, recoiled, sprung back into place, recovered its poise. Human interference had altered its circumstances, brutally, though intelligently and constructively, and in response that same 'heap' had spontaneously – *spontaneously* – resumed the ordinary business of being organised flesh. Knowing how it happens is not the same as knowing why it happens, and it seems to me that at a deep level we do not really know either why or how.

Other wonderful aspects of recovery appear within our embodied experience. What had become stale to us before falling ill can taste fresh again; neglected pleasures present themselves for reconsideration; we have the chance to make new resolutions (however fragile) about how we will make better use of our regained health and strength. All these good things are – or would be, did we not habitually forget them – the opportunities of ordinary embodied life. More particularly, they belong to those holding, as Sontag puts it, passports in the 'kingdom of the well';[14] by contrast they are just what are longed for by the sick. In his poem 'The Building', Larkin cruelly picks bare the hospital in-patient's longing for the free outside, with all its wonderful, reckless, humdrum ordinariness that is (seemingly) forever denied him[15]. In a less literal sense he is describing Rachel, too – not in hospital, but just as assuredly imprisoned by her diabetes, when an adult's caution prevents her from enjoying the treats of a school trip. At an alternative holiday camp for other diabetic children she would be one among many 'exactly like me ... I'll have a lot of fun and I'll be ordinary. Believe me, that would be the best thing of all.'

We have throughout been recalling the extraordinary wonderfulness of ordinary embodiment; but it has taken us some philosophical effort to do so. For those whose illness has deprived them of ordinary being, recalling it needs no such effort. The trouble lies in reclaiming it, and this – or as much of it as is possible – is treatment's aim.

EXISTENTIAL WONDER

That we are here at all

Whenever an individual patient receives treatment, that treatment is a response not merely to a given systemic (physiological, biochemical) disruption but to a disturbance in that remotely improbable material accident that constitutes each one of us. So is it not wonderful that we are here at all? Bill Bryson puts the point inimitably:

> For you to be here now trillions of drifting atoms had somehow to assemble in an intricate and curiously obliging manner to create you. It's an arrangement so specialized and particular that it has never been tried before and will only exist this once ... letting you experience the supremely agreeable but generally under-appreciated state known as existence. ... For all their devoted attention, your atoms don't actually care about you – indeed, don't even know that you are there. They don't even know that they are there. They are mindless particles, after all, and not even themselves alive. (... If you were to pick yourself apart with tweezers, one atom at a time, you would produce a mound of fine atomic dust, none of which had ever been alive but all of which had once been you.) Yet somehow for the period of your existence they will answer to a single rigid impulse: to keep you you.[16]

Both illness and treatment are – in different ways – organised disruptions to an existing 'arrangement' of atoms (only the agencies of disruption are different). Treatment is not conceived in these terms, of course, but nonetheless in material terms that is what it comes to.[(ii)] This uncomfortable equivalence is very present to Jen, who feels her body is 'letting her down' in response to treatment, notwithstanding that it is precisely because her body has (as it were) already 'let her down', in falling ill, that the treatment is being offered. The resemblance goes further: seeing how focused the nurses are 'made her realise, as nothing had, that the treatment was serious. Cancer was serious.' At some stages of her treatment, Jen will find illness and treatment partly indistinguishable. Both the cancer and the chemotherapy are organised disruptions to her body's patterns, and her atoms' arrangements.

Treatment is possible of course because (astoundingly) our 'arrangements' are patterned in ways so consistent that, as organisms, we can conform to a specification allowing us to come into the world, survive, beget offspring, and even come to a rudimentary understanding of what our patterns are meant to be and how they might be restored. In drawing on an

---

(ii) Here again, in this and the following two paragraphs, I express a number of points as I expressed them in Reference 3 (p. 134).

understanding of this conformity, the fact and success of treatment invites a further level of wonderment.

Yet still more wonderful is the accident (unless one's religious belief suggests otherwise) that at some level of increasing complexity amongst simpler, inert forms of matter an entirely new phenomenon emerges – consciousness, finding (so far as we know) its highest and perhaps only truly self-reflective form in embodied human nature. We are fantastically complex arrangements of very simple, very inert, parts. How mere complexity gives rise to the inner reality of sensation – let alone experience and self-reflection, and the ability to ponder questions of wonder – is as much a philosophical as it is a scientific mystery: perhaps more so. Treatment is ordinarily an intelligent, purposive, intentional and interpersonal activity. In the clinical consultation two intelligences – two emergences of intelligence from patterns of mere inert matter – jointly consider the problem that one of them has an altered experience. This is already astounding enough. But in treatment, they intervene in the pattern, in the 'arrangement', hoping thereby to intervene in the experience. In recognising this, we are drawn to further wonder. And in recognising *this* – this 'drawing to wonder' – we open the door to *ontological* wonder: wonder at ourselves, our agency and, indeed, our own capacity to wonder at all. Through our wondering, the otherwise material Universe wonders at itself; and heady though this thought may be, it suffuses the wonderfulness of treatment.

That we are capable of ecstasy and agony

The imagination is involved in ecstasy as much as in the agony of suffering. If we have led anything like an ordinarily fortunate life we will know at first hand most of the characteristic forms of sensory ecstasy, but we derive the fullest enjoyment of them through the imagination: anticipating, savouring, remembering them as well as – in effect – 'enduring' them. Like the minor irritants of an almost-comfortable posture that I described earlier, the ecstasies of the senses give the lie to Leriche's otherwise attractive view of health as 'life lived in the silence of the organs'. But they take their identity in contrast to the ordinariness of what plausibly *is* organic 'silence'. Ecstasy makes a pleasing poetic contrast with agony, but its *existential* contrast is with dull flatness, with tedium or with simply not noticing. Ecstasy is a special kind of noticing or attending, with always a small part of the attending being reflexive, turned back on itself, relishing the self-acknowledgement involved. In its way ecstasy involves a form of wonder because the imagination itself is an instance of what is wonderful, as well as the means through which we can recognise wonder. But – soberingly – this must also be true of suffering. The very root of wonder found in ecstasy has its baleful counterpart in the imaginative dimension of suffering: we are such creatures as cannot merely experience pain but be tormented by it in anticipating it, in abjuring it whilst undergoing it, and in remembering it even as we claw our way back out of it. Suffering involves a reflexive act of the imagination, something as regrettably worthy of wonder as ecstasy is ebulliently worthy.

In this sense, treatment often aims at transforming the content of the sensory provocations of our imaginations. Sadly treatment itself may, en route to perhaps a successful conclusion, provoke our imaginations adversely. Some of those undergoing chemotherapy suffer 'anticipatory vomiting' in the days or hours before a treatment cycle; the knowledge of what lies ahead is enough. Jen's imagination thrusts tuberculosis far deeper than cancer in its perceived threat to her, and only the seriousness of the treatment she is in fact to receive reveals the seriousness of the disease that she actually suffers. Poignantly, as we've seen, her imagination has also burdened the cosmetic provision of a wig with grievous symbolism.

Our existential 'metamorphosis'

We earlier reviewed the astounding metamorphic career of our physical forms, from conception to disintegration. It's of course matched – with due allowance for individual variations and cultural modifications – by the metamorphic career of our selves as agents. We begin and all-too-frequently end in helplessness, both physical and intellectual, though the resemblance perhaps stops there. The will-to-live that commands our infant bodies' growth – via our carers' attention – has a mordant echo in death-struggles, but there it will not strike others as having the same sense-making basis that nurtures the infant as such. But the will-to-live is for most of our lives obscured by the will-to-do, especially in such agent-centred contexts as liberal industrial societies.

Ask people when was the best time of their lives and they may well respond in terms of the period when they most felt they could act as they willed, when they most felt in control of their futures. Both in bodily and in spiritual terms, it is common for us to find a sense of invincibility in our prime – whenever we take that to be – replaced by doubt and scepticism as the next step in a relentless transition to what we may expect to be shocking vulnerability in decrepit age, and ultimate dissolution. Ignoring the intervening stages, how can it be possible that a will, an agency, can come into being from nothing; act for a while purposively and even (apparently) without impediment on life's stage; and then diminish into annihilation? The great actors of history may have shaped the world we live in today without the slightest possibility of their acting again in our own time. Some very few of us (as I write, former President Nelson Mandela continues to inspire even as he clings to life in intensive care) might move continents in their own lifetimes without the slightest prior basis in action before those lifetimes. At all levels of effect and power, human agency is somehow born of nothing and for a while simply cannot be repressed – it bristles and sparks and shoves almost unceasingly – and then it declines into extinction and, in most cases, oblivion as well.

A paler reflection of this, though in existential terms at least as terrible, is the rise and fall of cognition – one of agency's aspects in the ordinary case. Minds arise without antecedents, and minds disappear – mostly without trace. Is this not to be wondered at?

Treatment (for example, in addressing metabolic or psychotic disorders) can aim at adjusting the speed, the shape and, to an extent, the duration of this metamorphic career 'curve'; and this is wonderful enough in itself. But the basic framing of agency is beyond treatment's scope. Geoff's plight consists in part in the untimely loss of agency through his losing social awareness and interaction. One of the ironies of his treatment is that what it achieves – a 'lightening of mood' that is noticed, seemingly, only by the clinical staff at his nursing home – seems to benefit others rather than himself. His interactions with them have dwindled to little more than disturbances among his body's reactions of which he himself appears unaware. His 'existential metamorphosis' is prematurely complete.

WONDER IN PRACTICE

In this chapter I have tried to take wonder seriously as underlying and revealed in treatment: successful or otherwise, tolerable or otherwise, the very conception and ambition of treatment rests on (as well as intervenes in) the larger underlying wonder of human embodied experience. This does not exhaust the importance of wonder in clinical practice, however, and I will conclude with no more than a summary of some of its further 'supporting roles'. Each of these I think deserves further reflection beyond what I can attempt here.

Since the clinical encounter typically involves the two agencies, the two 'intelligences' as I earlier put it, of patient and clinician, it is convenient to let this review rest on their respective shoulders.

The clinician is first and foremost another embodied experiencing flesh, closely resembling the patient in virtually every important respect as regards the two large categories of 'bodily wonder' and 'existential wonder' under which I have considered our patients and their treatment. When the clinician addresses the patient's illness it is also her own mortality that she confronts; when she meddles in the patient's flesh, that flesh is also, in the final analysis, her own. This is easy to overlook and difficult to be mindful of; but one should be mindful of it nonetheless. Both the intimacy of this fleshly transaction, and the respect such intimacy demands, are *mutual* in character, and they demand that the intimacy be tempered by a kind of 'coolness', as Jane Macnaughton and I suggested in the previous Volume in this series.[17] The attitude of wonder involves both a preparative pause – before accepting the invitation to try to understand – and an implicit recognition of the limitations of the self and of one's own agency. Together these features of the attitude of wonder offer a good foundation upon which to build 'cool intimacy'.

The clinician also has to avoid complacency about either the general promise of a treatment or its application to an individual patient. Medical knowledge is at any one time provisionally adequate to a proportion of the questions that clinical practice throws up; but embodied human nature is enduringly complicated. The tenacity with which the desperately ill cling to life sometimes appears to suggest that nature is ineradicable; but we also know how fragile is our health and vigour. In undergoing treatment the patient risks disappointment or worse, and in the company of the clinician must submit himself to both the 'autonomy' of nature and the vagaries of circumstance. Treatments sometimes work and they sometimes fail, and (as is perhaps in Liz's mind when she ponders the 95% success rate of the procedure she has just undergone) the odds of success or failure are no more than a description of what is observed, statistically, over a dismayingly heterogeneous population. It is a matter of ontological wonder rooted in the consistency of our nature that, in the medium run, the aggregate numbers do come out right; but it may be a matter of moral wonder rooted in the lust for life that patients take their chances with toxic and uncertain treatments, hoping not to find themselves 'holding the wrong passports' when the numbers are counted.

In the end, perhaps our embodied natures – whether as patients or as clinicians – more strongly underpin, or constrain, the degree of our individual strength of will than we might like to suppose (or than is accounted for in the dominant place in so much healthcare ethical analysis that is occupied by an attachment to autonomy); for further exploration, *see* Iona Heath's chapter (Chapter 5) in this Volume. Notwithstanding, we persist in seeking, offering and taking treatments with all of their uncertainty. Our willingness to do so perhaps does not consciously echo the 'wonder of treatment' in the underlying sense that I have tried to explore in this chapter, but I think the willingness expresses that wonder, nonetheless.

REFERENCES

1 For instance: Evans M. Music, interrupted. In: Evans M., Ahlzén R., Heath I. and Macnaughton J., editors. *Medical Humanities Companion Volume One: symptom*. Oxford: Radcliffe Publishing; 2008. p. 19.

2 Leriche R., quoted in Canguilhem G. *On the Normal and the Pathological*. (Trans. C.R. Fawcett). New York, NY: Zone Books; 1991. p. 91.

3 Evans, H.M. Wonder and the clinical encounter. *Theoretical Medicine and Bioethics* 2012. **33**: 123–36. See p. 133.

4 Schopenhauer A. *The World as Will and Representation*. (Trans. E.F.J. Payne). Indian Hills, CO: The Falcon's Wing Press; 1958.

5 I am adapting the term from William Burroughs. Burroughs W.S. *The Soft Machine.* New York, NY: Grove Press; 1961.
6 Mann T. *The Magic Mountain.* (Trans. H.T. Lowe-Porter). London: Vintage Books; 1999. p. 276.
7 Gallagher S., Cole J. Body schema and body image in a deafferented subject. *Journal of Mind and Behavior.* 1995; **16**: 369–90.
8 Kant I. *Critique of Pure Reason.* (Trans. N. Kemp Smith). London: Macmillan Press; 1929. pp. 209 ff.
9 To echo a term of Wittgenstein's, albeit used in a very specific context and to a very specific purpose. Wittgenstein L. *Philosophical Investigations.* (Trans. G.E.M. Anscombe). Oxford: Blackwell; 1974. p. 218.
10 Diamond J., *C: because cowards get cancer too …*; London: Vermilion (Ebury Publishing); 1999.
11 Larkin P. The old fools. In: *High Windows.* London: Faber; 1974.
12 Magee B. *Confessions of a Philosopher.* London: Weidenfeld & Nicholson; 1997.
13 Macnaughton J. Seeing ourselves: interpreting the visual signs of illness. In Evans M., Ahlzén R., Heath I. and Macnaughton J., editors. *Medical Humanities Companion Volume One: symptom.* Oxford: Radcliffe Publishing; 2008. pp. 71–85.
14 Sontag S. *Illness as Metaphor.* New York, NY: Farrar, Strauss & Giroux; 1977. p. 3.
15 Larkin P. The building. In: *High Windows.* London: Faber; 1974.
16 Bryson B. *A Short History of Nearly Everything.* London: Black Swan; 2003. p. 1.
17 Evans M., Macnaughton J. Intimacy and distance in the clinical examination. In: Ahlzén R., Evans M., Louhiala P. and Puustinen R., editors. *Medical Humanities Companion Volume Two: diagnosis.* Oxford: Radcliffe Publishing; 2010. pp. 89–107; see pp. 96 ff.

3

Treatment – a matter between subjects

CARL EDVARD RUDEBECK

THE FRAMING OF TREATMENT

The origin

Medical treatment, whatever its specific features, is about the human condition in a complete sense, where biology and experience are inseparable but still distinct. Treatment originates in the situation where the suffering of one person calls for the action of another. From there it has grown into a major societal and scientific project. The origin of treatment has to be rediscovered in each individual situation to make the actions become therapeutic and not just instrumental. Treatment is what it is in a concrete sense, but it is also its own symbol, and here it reflects the idea of the dignity of human life. Layers of evidence, algorithms and imperatives have to be put aside in a gentle archaeological manoeuvre in order to grasp the original task. There is the moment, the room, a diagnosis and the two people establishing a patient–doctor relationship. And there may be ideas about what could be done to help the patient.

The process

Many treatments are singular. The problem is presented and the diagnosis stands out clearly enough to motivate a specific treatment, which may be anything from a word when distress, caused by worry, has been presented to a prescription of penicillin in a case of pneumonia. However, more often, the moment alone cannot fully contain the therapeutic needs. The beginning of diabetes is the opening of a life-long process that will involve many people. The moment extends into a relationship – people held in mutual awareness through time, and with openings into other relations.

The needs and the outcome

There are always outcomes of a therapeutic process. Some may be the very distinct changes in the biological body caused by its deliberate manipulation, and often enhanced by a placebo effect (or care effect; *see* Chapter 4) of varying degree. Others are more the outcomes of the process itself than of the particular aim of the treatment. These outcomes depend on the different needs that patients have besides becoming well, and how the doctor responds to these needs. Confirmation, reassurance, patient understanding and change in self-perception have been identified as such outcomes.[1] One can say that it is the patient's needs that ultimately set the frames for therapy. It is the patient who makes the doctor rather than the reverse. This founding fact is, however, easily concealed by a clinical worldview that limits to be a planned and knowledge-based intervention that has its effect on the patient. As much as treatment is embedded in its moral and symbolic implications, it is embedded in the facts of the therapeutic relation.

The patient

The subject of attributes

As an element of grammar, a 'subject' is that which is defined by its predicate, that is, its attributes, through which it may also relate to an object. The patient is a person who is ill and so justifiably treated. Illness and treatment are qualities of the members of the category named 'patients'. This is relevant when we talk about, and in other ways deal with, in the abstract, the predicament of the diseased. Medicine as theoretical knowledge is concerned with conceptualising and describing disease as accurately and specifically as possible. However, what in the abstract is a boundary between categories, is to the patient subject a situation of being cast out of the home of experienced health; of feeling that things are not the way that they should be.[2] The subject does not necessarily obey to its own linguistic categorisation in the way that it actually experiences itself and the world. Patient organisations, on the other hand, depend more on a generalisation of subjective experience, as their task is to harvest lobbying power from the various fates of their members. The distinction between the patient subject of attributes in medicine and of patient organisations on the one hand, and the individual, living subject on the other, reveals the inevitable ambiguity of language. Language loses its authority when it is believed to master experience, and it regains it only when it is understood to do no more than approaching it. It is exact only when the concepts are their own references, as in pure mathematics, but medicine is not mathematics, not even in its enthusiasm for measuring exercises. Physiology is life as mathematised, and, as such, it cannot do without approximations.

The cogito

The subject of attributes corresponds closely with the Cartesian cogito, the subject that *is* by virtue of its mental objects.[3] The subject–object relation of Cartesian rationalism turns into the form of existence of the subject. Accordingly, to the patient cogito, the symptoms are supposed to be the clear-cut and direct representations of what goes on in the body. Theoretical dualism is projected on individuals. In its knowing and thinking, the patient cogito gives the doctor the details of the symptoms, sticks to the prescriptions and reports the effects and side effects of treatment. Where the patient subject of attributes lends itself to discourses of various kinds, the cogito is the ideal patient for a humane and intellectualised medical practice. It is the pupil of clever patient education activities. Medicine really needs an abstract patient that is not only tied to disease but also stands for the lay perspective in the therapeutic relation, with which the medical can interact. The less that the doctor really knows the patient, the more the cogito tends to replace the individual and living patient, who then becomes involved in standard interactions and is exposed to standard information. This works well enough to keep medicine trustworthy in the eyes of society, but not to make patient-centredness superfluous as a distinct effort.[4] Gaps such as those between how doctors prescribe and how patients medicate, how doctors tell and how patients grasp, what doctors think is important and what patients find to be important, all reflect the confusion between the real and the ideal in clinical practice.

The patient cogito is a special case and a response to the need for medicine to be prepared for the encounter with the real patient. In a wider perspective, the cogito of the general 'other' is an assumption paving the way for any verbal exchanges whatsoever. You are never totally sure about the person with whom you talk – the other – or your own idea about the other, but nevertheless, you take her or his rational faculties for granted. Exchanging ideas is possible. Rationality is what makes human beings human. Descartes' cogito is not a logical judgement, but rather an attempt to give words to an individually lived insight, which once he had got it, he found to have general implications.[5]

The two abstract subjects are not contradictory but correspond to different faces of medicine. The patient's attributes – diseased and maybe helpless – tend to evoke paternalistic attention, which in its pure form includes a self-sufficiency of medicine in terms of interpretations and remedies. The cogito is treated with informed consent and through shared decision making to promote its autonomy. In the individual case, there is a mix, or balance, between these two, which is more or less appropriate. What decides the mix is out of the reach of the abstractions themselves. Concepts and theory disappear into the concreteness of the real-life situation. This is the life-world.[6] Experience that is governed by concepts has to be preceded by something else. By acknowledging this, phenomenology tries to rediscover the lost origin of knowledge. It may be a trap, but at least its grip helps avoid some of the most seductive delusions about the relation between experience and theory.

The subject as being

Medicine opens its doors to patients who bear the characteristics that warrant investigation and judgement. From the perspective of the healthcare organisation this is clear enough, but from the view of the patient it is very incomplete. The patient subject has a life before and outside of the abstraction. It is not any life, but the particular life of a specific patient. To accept such a premise you have to go one step further than trying to inject life into abstract concepts by stating that there is a human dimension to medicine that should not be forgotten. In his early essay 'Martin Heidegger and Ontology', Emmanuel Levinas, following Martin Heidegger, compares the subject – the cogito – of Western rationalistic and idealistic philosophy with the subject appearing in some of Plato's dialogues.[7] Whereas he finds that the first is defined by its non-temporal relations to objects, the second, the soul, 'is defined by *a mode of existence* that is inferior, by the fact of being involved with becoming, by finitude'. The subject is 'torn from the banquet of the Gods, and chained in the Cave'. Being subjected to finitude, the subject is not defined by *what* it is but by the fact *that* it is – that it exists. From the point of view of the subject, all relations are time relations. In Heidegger's thinking, human existence amounts to the understanding of being, which, however, is not an explicit understanding. Rather, being is hidden by the preoccupations of everyday life. Nonetheless, it is originally and always the possibility of its own authenticity in turning to itself as being.[8] The subject is being thrown into the world as its possibilities; existing is not primarily a matter of making judgements about the world, but of being thrown into it instant by instant. The world is a continuous temporal horizon from which it is impossible to escape. It is the facts. There is no future beside the facts and thus, in this respect, there is no choice other than the inescapable. The subject is also its own bodily facts and these are perhaps the most salient. In choosing itself in that which is given, the subject becomes the contingent unity of the world and an outlook on the world. 'The world is inseparable from the subject, but from a subject which is nothing but a project of the world, and the subject is inseparable from the world, but from a world which the subject itself projects.'[9]

Living the disease

One tends to live at a certain distance from the conditions that in a profound sense dictate life. Walking is just choosing a direction and walking off without questioning the neuromuscular physiology making it possible. Seeing is close to a constant forgetfulness of the eyes. The hands of one's watch just go round and round and do not point at the ultimate measure of lived time. Health holds its tongue. One dwells in the world, which keeps one busy. One knows that one lives but does not attend to the fact that one also knows that one knows that one lives. Every moment brings a possible space of clarity, where facts may be discerned and destiny disguised as partly written by oneself, but one falls out of that space more often than enduring it. This helps living on, but it also makes one's own life, except for its close at hand aspects, a returning stranger and surprise.

Falling ill undoes being as 'being as usual'. One's basic functions are revealed as they become malfunctions or dysfunctions. Depending on the intensity and severity, life itself may be put at stake. The vital role of that which is given and out of control becomes an intrusive insight. Out from that that one used to hold to be oneself stands the stubborn and menacing face of nature – an otherness deeper than identity. Through the expectations for the most immediate future – the protention – leads no other path than the unknown.[10] It is not just that the world is so much bigger than one's imagination, but that anything may be going on inside, beyond the fringe of awareness. The fact of being thrown into the world is demonstrated as the facts of biology.[11] This is of course not specific to the ill, but it is one major message of illness that the diseased cannot avoid hearing. Existence is laid bare, and the more ill one is, the more existence approaches the pure struggle of the body for its survival. When defining oneself as possibly needing treatment, intertwined with the hope of cure, is an existential need to live the disease. There are no alternatives to this, just as there are no escapes from the body that one is. Living the disease is not about taking on the sick-role; it induces questioning of some of the roles that one has already accepted within social life. Even common and non-threatening symptoms are in command of the perceptual field in the sense that they simply are there. In so far as one is temporarily forgetful of it, one is still only forgetful. The symptom is not gone for ever and this may be quite annoying since, with the distraction, hopes may rise that the symptom has actually vanished. Stubbornness is a key feature of a symptom and this distinguishes it from the profusion of transient noises of inner life. So living the disease is to live exactly that that one does not want to live. One needs what one does not want. The medical political discussion about the tension between wants and needs has here its reverse and it is stronger than any consumerist appeal. Disruption is primary. The American philosopher and physician Drew Leder calls it 'the hermeneutical moment'.[12] It strikes in silence and concealment while business seems to go on as usual. The anything from irritating to painful need to live one's facts is then realised within an inner dialogue, sometimes also involving close others, where the pros and cons of seeing a doctor are weighed against one another. Irrespective of the character of the ensuing decision, and of the actual course of the disease, the negotiation itself is the disclosure of being: 'This is in me – this is me – this is my near future.' Were it not inevitable, the negotiation would never have been undertaken. But the disclosure is still within an illusion of possible renunciation. As long as the signs of disease are not very obvious, even the intersubjectivity with close others is a homeland where wishes may challenge facts. Up until here disclosure is therefore only conditional.

The doctor

The subject of attributes

The doctor's path to the patient begins with the decision to become a doctor. By virtue of specific education, the attributes are attained that makes her or him a doctor: the accreditation, the title and the readiness to embark on the professional career. Attributes are discernible from the distance, so even if they are secondary to the contents of education, they are primary in the play of signals in society. Room is made in employment lists and healthcare facilities. People say: 'She is a doctor, a person who is prepared to be approached by patients by knowing about diseases.' The doctor subject is complementary to the patient subject. They share attributes, but that which the patient is, the doctor knows. The doctor's attributes are strong. They evoke expectations that may overrule the actual competence displayed. Here is a narcissist temptation of self-fulfilment through the attributes. If it dominates the professional self-image, this kind of self-fulfilment may only be counteracted by regulations against wrongdoing. Self-esteem stands against failure. The extreme doctor subject of attributes is the fake doctor, which is not just a fantasy.

But at the same time, the strength of the attributes is necessary and a blessing. The doctor not yet seen is important to people who struggle with symptoms and who negotiate their implications. This doctor is a horizon where self-control becomes conditional and, through this, important questions are raised. The doctor, not yet seen, is also the self-evident refuge and hope, in case vital self-functions seem to fail. The attribute is the symbol that works in culture. The doctor is owned, needed and feared. The task of the doctor of flesh and blood is to be worthy of this symbol.

The cogito

The doctor cogito is the aim of medical education. Aspirations are high regarding the amount, diversity and sophistication of knowledge. The mental representation that gradually, and depending on the philosophy laid down in the curriculum, orientates knowledge towards the task to be, and that thus ultimately defines the cogito, is the disease. Here the doctor exists by virtue of what is stored in consciousness, and by the ability to combine knowledge and make it operate in clinical situations. The life of the cogito is about knowing, and making judgements about reality – here the patient's symptoms and signs – from that which is known. Like the subjects of attributes, the doctor and patient cogitos preconceive each other. It takes both symptoms and knowledge to make a disease. Again, what the patient is the doctor knows. The hidden inner life of the patient's body, the network of billions of processes, where anything may happen at any time, is the home terrain of the doctor, chatting over the numeric results from laboratory tests and over magnetic resonance (MR) images. Here the range of the cogito touches the existential. The medical gaze looks straight into the fate of the patient. Science transcends itself into the brittle and powerful relation between patient and doctor.

The being a doctor

Being a doctor is belonging to a profession, bearing the attributes, knowing the facts, being prepared. In the absolute sense, the belonging is not tied to seeing patients. The just graduated doctor is a doctor who has not yet seen patients within the context of full professional responsibilities. But when meeting the first patient of his or her career, something becomes fulfilled. In that instant, being a doctor is also being as such. Attributes and knowledge pushes the doctor over the threshold of their own oblivion until the responsibility for the patient calls for standing back and reflecting over the next step to be taken, after which the life of the relationship again takes over. In this way, the encounter moves on in an interchange between involvement and detachment.[13] But what was seemingly primary – the professional role – turns into a secondary and reflective position. Involvement is first since it is a freedom before concepts within the limits set by the moral responsibility, but even these limits are the constituents of freedom in that they intuitively delineate the space of spontaneity.

Being a doctor, then, is to respond to the need of a patient through the relation. The attributes set the directions for how patient and doctor move into their common ground. Here they interact within the freedom given by the constraints of a medical encounter.

Treatment as mutual disclosure

Going to the doctor

In disease that follows its own course, it is the course that ultimately forms the decision to see a doctor, and this existential turn is the general form of 'the reason for encounter'. In the decision to approach a doctor the need to live the disease is disclosed. Every step from home to the doctor's office defies denial. It may be the last thing the patient wants to do and yet it is done. This confinement of autonomy is also the execution of it. The direction in geography denotes a vector of fate. The move is the message whatever the patient says when in the doctor's consulting room. The message is for both and so it is no longer private. It is embedded and it is clear enough. The patient may hesitate but the soil on the shoes from the walk does not. 'Here I am – there was no other way to go.'

The 'patient's delay' is about postponing the decision in a resistance to surrendering. In Anne Macleod's story, Jake will not accept his lot and he would rather stand the limitations it inflicts on him than be exposed to the felt humiliations of investigations. Maybe he has also realised that there is no really effective treatment available. He refrains from being a patient, although his attributes in terms of symptoms would clearly merit professional medical consideration. Even if he judges the odds for effective treatment correctly, there may still be a cost of staying on the healthy side of the entrance to the surgery.

Facing each other

Going to the doctor is itself the beginning of the process of treatment. It is self-care. Much is settled already there in the powers of the culturally anchored encounter. It works before it is executed, as a possibility and collective recognition of the recurring need of humankind to get its condition reflected in the attention of a doctor. Once facing each other, the patient does not ask the doctor for big words or gestures of compassion. He or she probably does not know what to ask about besides causes and cure, but embarking on a patient's journey is choosing what seems inescapable. The presence in face of each other is a fact and a disclosure that both patient and doctor live. But at the same time there is concealment. There has to be concealment. Existence, where self and time are one, is never a lasting experience or message. But it is always there as the subsumed and hidden relentlessness. The whole person is not an alternative to accept or reject for a doctor juggling with the pieces of the bio-psycho-neuro-endocrino-immuno-genetical disease model but a reality as demanding as the disease is to the patient. Paradoxically, therefore, the first step of treatment is responding to the patient's need to live the disease, even when, as is usually the case, this need is not overtly expressed. The patient seldom says, 'I want to be my disease.' Rather, there is hope or fear, or both, where the first is surpassing, and the second is being stuck in, the illness experience.

Facing each other is action. The doctor invites the patient into the consulting room by a signal, or by presenting his or her voice in a loudspeaker or by actually collecting the patient from the waiting room. The potential becomes real and values are at stake. The cultural investment has been made at the cost of disclosure. Something is, but still it is something only if it is preceding something else. It is a stand-still, where the interior of the premises and the bodies of other patients fade into the background while the relationship takes its first shape of non-fulfilment, but a stand-still that also falls forward and vanishes into its own future behind the door.

This moment, repeating itself through tens of thousands of times in the routine of the life of a doctor, is also the constant appointment of the doctor to be a doctor and not just being the bearer of professional attributes. The call is the patient's disclosure through being there, having moved from then to now, from there to here. The origin of treatment is accepting this call from which there is no escape. In conforming to the code of a medical encounter, and in giving in to the expectations that the patient does not want to have but nevertheless has, the doctor sees to it that the patient is no longer totally at a loss. What happens here, in the midst of rush and routines, and thus concealed within itself, if things turn out well, as they often do, is the confluence of the patient's need to live the disease and the doctor's need to be a doctor. They are exposed to each other, and in just being so, for a moment, their relation finds its resonance in a stage management beyond their own reach. A foundation for treatment is laid that itself is therapeutic.[14]

Telling and asking

Having accepted his or her appointment, the doctor's office is in itself an offer and a challenge to the patient. Important and unusual things are said and are welcomed. 'Tell me!' In many of the conversations of everyday life, people hide behind what they say. Language is for demonstrating conformity and for belonging. The burning facts are exactly those that are not pronounced. In the consulting room the opposite order prevails. Time is quite short, and there is no room for prevarication. The attention of both patient and doctor is on the experience of the former that quite often resists description. Words are only the far approximations of the experiences. On top of this is the deep ambivalence of being exposed to the vulnerability and limitation that life is. If the symptom is really threatening, ambivalence is touched or overrun by fear. With minor ailments, the overt drama may be no more than irritation, but still one's routines have been sacrificed, and what if the doctor sends the message that this was an unnecessary visit (that one of course in one sense wants it to be)? The symptom presentation is a speech act that in overcoming its resistance gets its full articulation in incompleteness. In the empty and silent moments listening does not stop. The patient hears, through his or her own telling and perhaps for the first time, how things really are. In hearing oneself, there are also the doctor's senses and attention. Saying and sharing are the same, as are the personal and the common, as are saying and living, as are listening and living. The symptom presentation is a moment of disclosure within a deepened intersubjectivity. Differing from the negotiation preceding the walk to the doctor, here the experience becomes definite. Conditionality remains, however, on the level of actions. Patient and doctor are still within the consultation of the consultation, where the doctor is consulted about the problem and the patient still has control. The telling includes, or is followed by, a request for advice. The disclosure does not mean giving up responsibility. Rather it is taking it. Facing the facts of one's own predicament in the sequence of acts from then until now is living as taking responsibility. In this situation the doctor has the great and delicate responsibility to help the patient to stay in the position of deciding. The dynamics of the disclosure, both parties being moved by life in its openness, tends to hasten them past the patient's first possible gain of the consultation, which is a widened view on his or her own situation. However serious the condition may seem, the decision to proceed in the way suggested by the doctor is ultimately with the patient. The doctor's task is to stay sufficiently close to and steady enough for the patient to dare to make the decision. The imperatives of guidelines and rules of action are not for the patient, but only their rationale as translated through the doctor's moral involvement.

The consultation of the consultation is not just a single and specific situation. In the lasting patient–doctor relation it is a room for the exchange of experience and information, for mutual consideration and continuous balancing of responsibility. Here the inexorable facts become the patient's choices through which life is again mastered. When, in this volume, we meet Rachel, the young girl with diabetes portrayed by Anne Macleod, there is no doctor close. The doctors seeing her and her mother in the hospital visits are anonymous cogitos. The one doctor with a name, Dr Friend, swings his attribute pen to help Rachel get a permit to join the class trip, but Rachel's medical companion in disease is the nurse Dax, who trains and coaches Rachel to take as much control as possible. The person who never consults, but who stays frightened on the surface of what has really happened, is Rachel's mother. Her attention is directed to the laboratory tests and to behaving well, and she has no faith in her daughter's developing abilities to handle the technicalities of diabetes. Still Rachel really needs her mother in living her disease and in facing the inescapable. She cannot take the full view of a grown-up; the sadness and hope of an existential re-orientation, and in so far as this is unattainable for her mother, Rachel will not get the chance to cry out her desolation and to get it confirmed and contained in her mother's lap. Here could be the honest moments, when love and sense for realities may have seeded plants of self-respect in a girl who will soon embark on the unpredictable trajectory of a teenager.

Giving in

There is a boundary between self and other even within oneself. From the otherness, which is the self as disintegrated, nature claims its sovereignty. The boundary extends into the consultation. Here, otherness is the competence of the doctor, whose knowledge may penetrate every layer of skin and integrity of the patient to take a view of what may be going on inside. The doctor may suggest exactly this to the consulting patient. The doctor believes that the problem is out of the patient's control, and that it may be good to intervene. In trust, the patient may decide to pass the boundary. This may give peace. The patient, subjected to his or her own facts, becomes a subject in making itself available to the acts and actions of treatment and so in accepting to be the object of treatment. This is literally living the disease through living the inescapable. Accepting anaesthesia, lying still for the necessary time and facing probable post-operative pain are all very active decisions and acts, but they are hidden within that that is expected. So, stating that being a subject is by being an object is not a play with words. It brings out something quite vital about medicine. The objectifying gaze focused on the patient is often the prerequisite for the doctor to act in the interest of the patient subject. The reason as to why a humanistic critique often still targets the 'objectivism' of medicine is that the object too often occupies almost all attention, reducing the person subject to an adding or a memento. The ethos of medicine is found to be buried in its procedures. However, with the critique goes a slightly contemptuous connotation of the word 'object', which renders the understanding of medicine stuck in a simplistic subject–object dichotomy. The roles of the play are frozen before it starts. The patient subject, who lives his or her own facts by choosing to be an object in the hands of medicine, embraces the dichotomy without disappearing into it, which is not to say that it is an easy passage. But while the patient decides to be an object, the doctor recognises the subject through all stages of treatment. This is a matter of recognition by being faithful. The covered, tube-connected and sleeping patient subject is the law of the operating theatre. The breathing, even when assisted, is human.

Liz is reluctant and scared all the way through. The cell-changes belong to the dim outskirts of her life in a mix of estrangement and embarrassment. The eventuality of cancer makes her, in fact, fight for her life in the pink environment, while the receptionists, nurses and doctors barely see more than their routines. She is left alone in the hurried correctness of the treating doctor with the nurse making noises in the background. When treated like an object it becomes much more difficult to be one. The only thing that saves Liz is her choice to be there, encouraged and advised by a doctor whom she knows. She placed herself into the smell of her own body during diathermy.

Being given in

Rachel had no consultation at the debut of her disease, which was her story in Volume One. She was then in an emergency state. Later, and under the guidance of Dax, she takes the first steps towards autonomy, at least in terms of management. With time, it is to be hoped that she will claim room for consulting even within the scheduled minutes of the doctor's visits.

When limited in expressing oneself, as is Geoff, or in comprehending the disease and its implications, as is Geoff's wife Jen, negotiating and deciding about becoming an object of treatment is no longer possible. They both easily become objectified, in a definite way, through their diseases, and have very little influence over what is decided for them. This leads to a certain loneliness on behalf of both parties of the patient–doctor relation but the only one who can change this is the doctor. The relation needs to be discovered as a lived reality. Only when close and touched, and when appointed a doctor by the disclosed existence of the other, alternatives may be considered in an ethically and professionally reasonable way.[15] We do not see much of this in the tragedy of Jen and Geoff, a tragedy that is far from unique. It is possible that there may have been instants where a doctor, sitting on a chair opposite to one of them, embodied seeing and compassion. If this is the case, it is still not possible to tell how this would have changed the decisions about treatment. In formal terms they may not have changed at all. In terms of dignity, however, the gap between them would be infinite.

Concluding remark – spurious authenticity

Existence is all there is and yet it is fugitive. It disappears into its resemblances, hidings and proxies in 'unbearable lightness'.[16] It discloses itself as otherness in the midst of the familiar; breaks through as clear sightedness when consciousness is all involved in living as it is. Mostly life goes on in more modest moods and in the repeating of the seemingly necessary in a permanent loss of authenticity.[17] This may nourish an idealisation of authenticity, the lost treasure of humanness. To the diseased, authenticity is harsh. Living is being subjected to limitations, suffering and finitude and the search for mitigation and escape is very reasonable. In spite of this, the thesis of this chapter is that the patient needs to live that that is sensed in authenticity, but the term preferred within the text is 'disclosure', as the connotations of the latter are more factual than valuing. The doctor may promote or provoke disclosure as an intersubjective event, but only if responding to the call from the patient. This may appear quite striking but in fact it is hardly noticed other than as a moment of mutuality. This friendship over human suffering, where its uneven distribution in favour of the doctor is only temporary, is a given and is therefore passive.[18] The deed is to let it happen. Therefore, disclosure is never a success, but the sentimentality of the doctor may be mistaken for disclosure. Here a trend may be lying in waiting, and if advancing, doctors will be challenged by the tyranny of a spurious authenticity.

REFERENCES

1 Andén A, Andersson S-O, Rudebeck CE. Satisfaction is not all – patients' perceptions of outcome of general practice consultations, a qualitative study. *BMC Fam Pract.* 2005 Oct 24; **6**: 43.

2 Svenaeus F. *The Hermeneutics of Medicine and the Phenomenology of Health: steps towards a philosophy of health practice* [thesis]. Linköping: Studies in art and sciences – Department of health and society; 2000.
3 Levinas E. Martin Heidegger and ontology. *Diacritics*. 1996; **1**(spring): 11–32. (Trans. Committee of Public Safety).
4 Stewart M, Belle Brown J, Weston WW, *et al. Patient-centered Medicine: transforming the clinical method*. Oxford: Radcliffe Publishing; 2003.
5 Husserl E. *The Crisis of European Sciences and Transcendental Phenomenology*. (Trans. D Carr). Evanston: Northwestern University Press; 1970. pp. 75–8.
6 Husserl E, op. cit., pp. 103–86.
7 Levinas E, op. cit.
8 Heidegger M. *Being and Time*. (Trans John Macquarrie and Edward Robinson). Oxford: Basil Blackwell; 1962. pp. 219–24.
9 Merleau-Ponty M. *Phenomenology of Perception*. London: Routledge & Kegan Paul; 1962; p. 430.
10 Husserl E, op. cit., pp. 168–9.
11 Heidegger M, op. cit.
12 Leder D. *The Absent Body*. Chicago, ILL: Chicago University Press; 1990. p. 78.
13 McWhinney IR. Being a general practitioner: what it means. *Euro J Gen Pract*. 2000; **6**: 135–9.
14 Ridd M, Shaw A, Lewis G, *et al*. The patient–doctor relationship: a synthesis of the qualitative literature on patients' perspectives. *Br J Gen Pract*. 2009; **59**(561): 268–75.
15 Nortvedt P. Sensibility and clinical understanding. *Med Health Care and Philos*. 2008; **11**: 209–19.
16 Kundera M. *The Unbearable Lightness of Being*. New York, NY: HarperCollins Publishers; 2008.
17 Heidegger M, op. cit.
18 Nortvedt P, op. cit.

4

Deciding on treatment

PEKKA LOUHIALA

> Those who rely on experience alone are accordingly called empiricists. Similarly, those who rely on reason are called rationalists. And these are the two primary sects in medicine. The one proceeds by means of experience to the discovery of medicines, the other by means of indication.[1]

> Yet physicians, in their treatment, often have to take account of the so-called influence of the moral over the physical, and also of any number of family and social considerations which have nothing to do with science.

> Compassion and blind empiricism are the prime movers of medicine; later came reflection bringing doubt, then scientific verification.[2]

Most of us have at least some experiences of pain, as well as at least some experiences of the relief that pain medication can give in such situations. It may come as a surprise, then, that painkillers have in most cases *not* been tested according to the strict standards of contemporary clinical research. That a patient reports having been helped is the weakest kind of evidence or no evidence at all to support the effect of a treatment – at least according to current mainstream medical thinking.

If the patients cannot be trusted, how do physicians decide about treatments? Is clinical medicine as scientific as it at least tacitly claims to be – and patients seem tacitly to believe? In general, what are the roles of science, experience and values in clinical decision making? In particular, what is this thing called *evidence* that suddenly appeared in the medical vocabulary in the early 1990s? Let us look at this question first in the stories of our patients.

Rachel has been on insulin therapy since the initial diagnosis of juvenile diabetes. What is the evidence for this treatment? After all – and it is somewhat surprising – no randomised controlled trials (RCTs) have been performed on insulin in that condition. Of course, nobody would suggest a placebo-controlled trial of insulin treatment for diabetes today. The survival of the first ever diabetic treated with insulin – together with the millions to follow – was hard enough evidence. In addition to insulin therapy, Rachel is also receiving much else, none of which has the support of evidence that is ranked high in the common hierarchies of clinical evidence. The general experience of diabetics of her diabetes nurse as well as her particular experience of Rachel (and Rachel's mother) are crucial in the daily decisions concerning insulin doses, diet and exercise.

Jake, on the other hand, has no definitive diagnosis yet. His symptoms and the initial assessment by Dr Siddha (*see* Volume 2 in this series) suggested irritable bowel syndrome (IBS), and Jake has tried peppermint oil as Dr Siddha advised. In this case, placebo-controlled RCTs exist and they show that the number needed to treat (NNT) for peppermint oil in IBS is 2.5 (that is, a number of two or three patients need to be treated in order to benefit one of them).[3] The oil seemed to 'help a bit' when Jake took it, but he continued to have symptoms that were not mild. Jake did not want further diagnostic testing, however, and we can only guess why.

The appointment between Liz and Dr Patience can perhaps be regarded as successful if the technical procedure is considered in isolation. When the experiences of the patient are added, however, the picture is different. We are told, 'The nurse looked at her coldly, and the eponymous Dr Patience did not live up to her name.' A procedure called LLETZ (large loop excision of the transformation zone) was performed on her, but the meaning of the abbreviation was never explained to Liz.

Geoff, in turn, has been evaluated at a geriatric unit, the Hope Ward. After suffering a stroke he has been dependent on his wife, and he is now suffering from depression. We learn that he 'stared resolutely out the window, did not look or speak – not once – throughout the full half hour they sat there'. However, according to Ward Sister Merchant, the antidepressants are beginning to work and a change for the better has been seen in the last few days. A discharge from the ward is planned and Jen, his poor wife, does not seem to understand how unrealistic the plan is. It is difficult to know the exact role of antidepressant medication in this case, but even then it is clear that it is a small piece in the puzzle when Geoff's future treatment is planned.

This chapter consists of two parts. The first part examines the relevance of evidence-based medicine (EBM) to these problems. The second part looks beyond quantitative evidence and examines other components of clinical decision making.

GOODBYE EVIDENCE-BASED MEDICINE

My personal acquaintance with EBM began in the mid-1990s, when our medical faculty decided to offer EBM courses for medical students. Before that, our staff had to be trained to be able to deliver the courses, and many of us attended a two-day training course on the basics of EBM. The teachers were very enthusiastic about the topic and their enthusiasm took a hold on me. 'This is really something new,' I thought. 'Now I have the tools to find out the truth.'

After the course I decided to apply my new skills to a frequent clinical problem from my paediatric practice. I chose *molluscum contagiosum*, a benign, common viral skin infection, which usually resolves within months. Parents, however, are often worried about the condition. Using my freshly acquired skills I managed to locate two RCTs on the topic.

The results were disappointing. One of the trials showed no effect at all, and, in the other, a potentially highly toxic substance, podophyllotoxin, was used on teenagers rather than young children. The search did not bring anything useful for my practice. As with all love affairs, I began with unrealistic expectations and my honeymoon with EBM was soon over.

The philosophical origins of EBM extend to at least the early 19th century, when Thomas Beddoes in England proposed the systematic collection and indexing of medical facts, and Pierre Louis in France led a movement called 'Médecine d'Observation'.[4,5] According to Louis, '[P]hysicians should not rely on speculation and theory about causes of disease, nor on single experiences, but they should make large series of observations and derive numerical summaries, from which real truth about the actual treatment of patients will emerge.'[6]

The direct antecedent of the EBM movement of the 1990s was the work of Archie Cochrane two decades earlier. Cochrane argued that too many interventions of dubious or unknown safety and efficacy were used in medicine, and that these interventions caused harm at both individual and population levels through iatrogenic injury, waste of resources and failure to take up more effective treatments.[7] Another antecedent of EBM was the discipline called clinical epidemiology, which was developed in the 1980s.

The concept of EBM was introduced for the first time in *The Journal of the American Medical Association* (*JAMA*) in 1992.[8] A specific definition was not given, but EBM was characterised as de-emphasising intuition, unsystematic clinical experience or reasoning based on changes in normal bodily functions as sufficient grounds for clinical decision making. Initially, the goal was obviously to minimise the use of non-evidentiary knowledge and reasoning in clinical practice.[9] A few years later, a broader definition was provided:

> Evidence-based medicine ... is the conscientious, explicit and judicious use of current best evidence in making decisions about the medical care of individual patients.[10]

As years passed, even broader definitions were suggested:

> EBM is currently understood to incorporate clinical epidemiological data, meaningful deliberations of professionals' pathophysiological knowledge and clinical experience, together with patient preferences.[11]

> [T]he evidence to which EBM refers to ought to comprise six dimensions: scientific evidence, theoretic evidence, practical evidence, expert evidence, judicial evidence and ethics-based evidence.[12]

But what *is* EBM really and does it differ from the clinical medicine that was practised before its introduction? A quick look at the literature makes it easy to agree with Timmermans and Mauck, who note that the term:

> is loosely used and can refer to anything from conducting a statistical meta-analysis of accumulated research, to promoting randomized clinical trials, to supporting uniform reporting styles for research, to a personal orientation toward critical self-evaluation.[13]

The problem with the definitions of EBM is that they are so general and vague that they do not provide a *demarcation line* between EBM and non-EBM. As Tonelli[14] notes, there is certainly not a physician alive who would not claim to practise EBM if it is defined as 'the conscientious, explicit and judicious use of current best evidence in making decisions about the medical care of individual patients'.

In spite of the demarcation problem, EBM received huge attention from the medical community and editors of leading medical journals within the years after its introduction; indeed a journal *Evidence-Based Medicine* was launched in 1995. In the somewhat sarcastic words of Feinstein and Horwitz, EBM 'acquired the kind of sanctity [that is] often accorded to motherhood, home, and the flag'.[15] EBM was welcomed most enthusiastically in the United Kingdom, possibly because 'its ideology is largely a simple form of Enlightenment rationalism: following Leibniz and Bacon, the idea is to resolve differences through measurement, calculation and comparison'.[16]

Critical voices were, however, soon heard. A philosopher of medicine wondered why basing clinical decisions upon evidence was thought to be either new or exciting and, according to himself, he also pondered anxiously 'what it was that clinical decisions used to be based on before this big idea'.[17] Several physician-authors pointed out that important aspects of clinical medicine were overlooked by focusing on the results of clinical research.[18]

Only six years after the introduction of the concept, Charlton and Miles published a paper entitled 'The rise and fall of EBM'.[19] Recently, Tonelli[20] went as far as arguing that 'it is time to remove evidence, both term and notion, from clinical decision making, for it no longer serves any useful purpose, if it ever did'.

Critique

In general, criticism has concerned the claimed novelty of the approach, the emphasis on randomised trials, the proposed hierarchy of evidence and the role of individual practising physicians.

First, the original EBM working group initially made the claim that EBM presented a new *paradigm* in clinical medicine. The bold claim has been repeated numerous times,[21] but it has never been properly scrutinised. If it were true, it would imply that something very fundamental changed and that medicine practised before EBM was highly questionable.

It is enough to look at Thomas Kuhn's original writing to demonstrate that EBM can by no means be considered a new paradigm in clinical medicine. In the postscript accompanying the second edition of *The Structure of Scientific Revolutions*, Kuhn notes that in much of the original text the term 'paradigm' was used in two different senses. In the first, wider sense, paradigms refer 'to the entire constellation of beliefs, values, techniques, and so on shared by the members of a given community', and, in the second, narrower sense, they denote concrete puzzle-solutions or *exemplars* in a field of established science.[22] It is obvious that EBM is not a new paradigm of clinical medicine in any of these meanings.

Second, in the early years of EBM, in particular, randomised trials and meta-analyses were seen as the gold standard and evidence from other kinds of studies was almost entirely neglected.[23] A textbook on EBM was explicit on this: 'If you find that the study was not randomized, we'd suggest that you stop reading it and go on to the next article. Only if you can't find any randomized trials should you come back and have another go at it.' [24] All of this happened in spite of the fact that one of the founding fathers of RCTs, Sir Austin Bradford Hill, had already remarked in 1966 that

> [t]he history of science, however, shows that frequently with a new discovery, a new technique, or a new theory of disease, the pendulum at first swings too far. Has this been so with the controlled trial? Is it true, as Cromie (1963) has suggested, that 'little or no credence is now given to clinical observations even by experienced investigators' while there is 'a blind acceptance of double-blind trials without a critical evaluation of their short-comings and their ability to mislead as well as to lead'. ... Any belief that the controlled trial is the only way would mean not that the pendulum had swung too far but that it had come right off its hook.[25]

There are several pitfalls with the RCT approach. The evidence gained from RCTs is skewed and biased towards therapeutic rather than preventive interventions, and towards simple pharmacological rather than complex behavioural and/or social care.[26] The conclusions of an RCT refer to an average patient who fulfilled the criteria for admission. In fact, RCTs were transferred to clinical medicine from agricultural research and they were originally not intended to answer questions about individual patients.[27] In addition, there are numerous situations in which clinical decisions depend on individual pathophysiology, not published evidence. Examples of such situations are mechanical ventilation, blood transfusion and electrolyte alterations.

After the early enthusiasm of the EBM movement, the limits of quantitative approaches in general and RCTs in particular were highlighted in the *British Medical Journal* (*BMJ*), the same journal that had a central role in the creation of EBM.

> Doctors have traditionally placed high value on numerical data, which may in reality be misleading, reductionist, and irrelevant to the real issues. The increasing popularity of qualitative research in the biomedical sciences has arisen largely because quantitative methods provided either no answers or the wrong answers to important questions in both clinical care and service delivery.[28]

> However, in the context of the debate about evidence based medicine, it is vital to reiterate that good 'evidence' goes further than the results of metaanalysis of randomised controlled trials. The limitations of these trials, and the evidence about barriers to their utilisation by practitioners, should not lead to cynicism about the role of research evidence in health care. We need to be sure that it is the right kind of research to answer the questions posed.[29]

Third, the hierarchical approach to evidence that has been adopted by EBM and clinical guidelines is problematic. Since the first published hierarchy of evidence in the 1970s, numerous different classifications, usually of increasing elaboration and complexity, have appeared, and they all place RCTs at the highest level.[30]

Evidence from RCTs is, however, not necessarily better or stronger than evidence from other types of research, for example, observational studies, pathophysiology or even a single case study. Three examples demonstrate this. First, type 1 diabetes was always fatal until insulin was available. It is hard to imagine more powerful evidence than the survival of the first patient who received insulin.

Second, the evidence of a causal link between smoking and lung cancer is not questioned (except by lobbyists of the tobacco industry) although no RCTs exist.

Third, Poynard *et al.*[31] have shown that conclusions based on 'good' methodology had no clear survival advantage over methodology that is ranked lower in the standard hierarchies. The main problem with the hierarchical approach to evidence is that it attempts to rank research methods that are incommensurable. Experiments, observations and theoretical thinking are all needed in building up the evidence base for clinical medicine. Sir Michael Rawlins elegantly summarised the importance of all of these aspects:

> For those with lingering doubts about the nature of evidence itself I remind them that while Gregor Mendel (1822–84) developed the monogenic theory of inheritance on the basis of experimentation, Charles Darwin (1809–82) conceived the theory of evolution as a result of close observation, and Albert Einstein's (1879–1955) special theory of relativity was a mathematical description of certain aspects of the world around us. William Harvey's discovery of the circulation of the blood—as he described in *De Motu Cordis*—was based on an elegant synthesis of all three forms of evidence.[32]

Fourth, the initial ideal that all clinicians should have the time, skill and motivation to conduct their own searches and critical appraisals may be unrealistic. A working group on ethics and EBM concluded that

> it remains debatable, however, whether a practising doctor should have methodological training to the extent that he or she can independently assess the value of research reports. The basic goal for education in this regard, should be to promote a critical attitude toward all evidence claims, including those from the EBM movement.[33]

An individual clinician cannot be independent and self-reliant, not even in his or her own field of specialisation. John Hardwig has emphasised the 'climate of trust' that is required to support much of our knowledge:

> In most disciplines, those who do not trust cannot know; those who do not trust cannot have the best evidence for their beliefs. In an important sense, then, trust is often epistemologically even more basic than empirical data or logical arguments: the data and the argument are available only through trust.[34]

The existence of a journal called *Evidence-Based Medicine* is a tacit admission that the goal of individually practised EBM is perhaps not attainable.[35] Another example of a new authority is 'the prestigious Cochrane Collaboration', which is often cited in the news as a source of reliable evidence on medical issues. As long ago as 1997 Feinstein and Horwitz noted in their sarcastic style that '[a] new form of dogmatic authoritarianism may then be revived in modern medicine, but the pronouncements will come from Cochranian Oxford rather than Galenic Rome'.[36]

Not the baby with the bath water

In revolutions, partisans on all sides have an interest in making matters seem simpler than they really are.[37] The critics of EBM go too far when they say that 'evidence-based medicine (EBM) is a powerful instrument in objectifying the world, annihilating the subject, and eroding clinical freedom'.[38] On the other hand, the proponents, too, exaggerate when they argue that '[e]vidence-based medicine (EBM) has had enormous impact on clinical medicine',[39] or, that '[t]he ideology of evidence-based medicine (EBM) has dramatically altered the way we think, conceptualize, philosophize and practice medicine'.[40]

Notwithstanding the conceptual problems, the EBM movement has, however, had at least a modest positive impact on medical education and clinical practice. Medical students of today are taught scepticism towards anecdotal evidence, and they are given tools for critical thinking and critical reading of scientific papers. The tools were there already, but it took EBM to bring them to the desks of practising clinicians.

Charlton and Miles declared in 1998 that 'the time is ripe for the "evidence-based" mantra to be silenced and dissenting voices to be heard'.[41] More than 10 years after that the term 'EBM' is still alive but the world is not as black and white as it was in the 1990s. The term is, however, still used loosely and the unnecessary tensions around it have not vanished. Why not keep the good things and give up the controversial term altogether?

WHAT ELSE IS THERE?

The 'evidence' in EBM refers to evidence from *scientific studies*, although this has seldom been explicitly stated. The nature of the 'science' behind those studies has not been questioned except by rare observers from outside. One of those observers argued that

> evidence-based practices maintain an antiquated understanding of evidence as "facts" about the world in the assumption that scientific beliefs stand or fall in light of evidence. This understanding of evidence is explicitly positivist, and such a picture of science has been seriously undermined by post-positivist philosophies of science.[42]

This positivist view is attractive to many, because it seems to rationalise the complex process of clinical reasoning. It does so, however, by eliminating from consideration culture, contexts and the subjects of knowledge production.[43]

No one denies that scientific evidence is an essential part of clinical reasoning but there is much more to the picture. Like love in the famous song, evidence is a 'many-splendored thing', and the sort of evidence we think worth looking for depends on the sort of question that we want to be answered.[44] In addition to scientific evidence, at least *moral, aesthetic, juridical* and *economic* evidence can influence clinical judgements in patient care.

The following figure shows some components of treatment decisions. It is not exhaustive but it demonstrates the complexity of the situation and the interplay of scientific evidence, experience and values on both the physician's side and the patient's side of the diagram. In other words, it demonstrates that there are many kinds of evidence in addition to the common understanding of the word in the context of EBM. Even minor changes in any of the variables may affect the final decision. The figure also demonstrates the interplay between the general and the particular: knowledge and experience of *this* patient is as essential as general knowledge and experience. No amount of empirical data can ever tell us what we ought to do in a particular situation.[45]

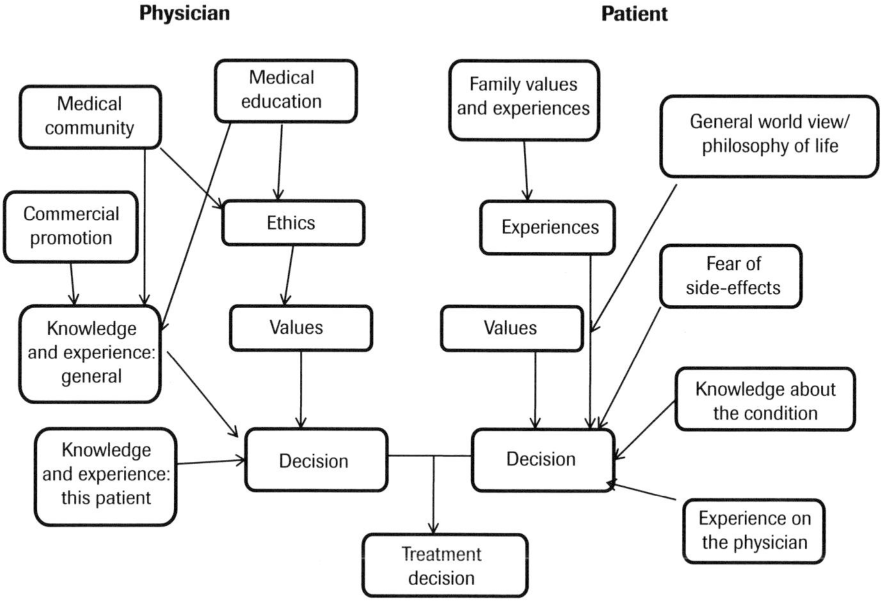

Figure 4.1 Some determinants of a treatment decision (modified from[46])

Values

Whatever the evidence we have for or against a treatment, every decision includes value judgements. Numbers are only numbers and, as such, they only advise and do not dictate. Even ethicists sometimes don't see this.

> Either the evidence is valid, in which case you must attend to it; or it is not, in which case you have to act based on some sort of reason; or you just do not know, but need to decide on a course of action nonetheless. 'Art' will not help you here – neither hunches, guesses nor intuition.[47]

The citation reveals a common misunderstanding that seems to resemble the *naturalistic fallacy* or *is-ought problem*. Although Goodman seems to claim otherwise, there is no compelling reason for the clinician to act in one direction or another, *whatever* the evidence is. Clinical evidence is *probabilistic* by nature and a treatment decision calls for a value judgement in any case.

The central role of values does not imply, however, that value conflicts are common. On the contrary, in the vast majority of cases the value worlds of physicians and patients overlap quite sufficiently, and no conflicts arise.

The values behind a treatment decision are often hidden and implicit, but that does not mean that they are less important. Openly expressed values make the process transparent, but hidden values obscure it, particularly in cases where there are value conflicts. The following examples demonstrate the role that values play in clinical situations where a superficial examination would not reveal any major role.

In the first example, patients with an abdominal aortic aneurysm and their surgeons were studied during the process of deciding which treatment was necessary. Initially, the research team planned to develop a brochure first and to start empirical research on patient autonomy afterwards. The hypothesis of the study was that individualised evidence-based decision support could empower patients to take part in the decision-making process together with the surgeon and thus would encourage patients to become more autonomous.[48]

However, during the process of translating the results of the decision model into an actual brochure, the researchers became aware that there are many different ways to produce and present 'evidence-based' facts. Choosing between them seemed to require certain normative and moral values. Different choices in the process of producing and presenting facts also appeared to lead to different moral consequences, in particular regarding patient autonomy. Molewijk *et al.*[49] concluded their findings about 'scientific facts' as follows:

> Many patients and physicians consider scientific facts to be true, objective and value-neutral. However, these so-called facts are not as hard as they appear. In fact they emerge from a black box: the facts have travelled a long, hidden and sometimes arbitrary journey before they are presented as "the facts."

The second example concerns the treatment of middle ear infection (acute otitis media (AOM)), a very common disease in childhood. Perhaps surprisingly, the treatment decision contains several value judgements.[50]

If the diagnosis is certain, the first question seems to be whether the patient needs antibiotics or not. Different medical traditions offer different answers, and none of them can claim to be superior to others. In many countries, the patient would receive antibiotics but in the Netherlands, for example, the family doctor may well choose the 'wait-and-see' option.

Of course, there is a vast amount of research – and evidence – on AOM but the problem is that the evidence does not help a lot. According to one meta-analysis, seven children have to be treated with antibiotics for one to benefit; according to another meta-analysis, the number is 17. The problem is that no one can tell in advance who is going to be the lucky patient.

If the physician decides to prescribe antibiotics for the child, there are still value judgements to be made. Which of the many possible antibiotics should be given? Do price, taste, number of daily doses, length of the course or spectrum covered by the drug matter? If every dose means a struggle between the child and his or her parents, it may be that the latter would prefer a single daily dose for three days to a twice daily dose for a week. When deciding about the spectrum of the drug, the doctor has to balance the interests of the patient and the society in general: a liberal use of wide-spectrum antibiotics will very probably be harmful for many *future* patients.

There are other issues about treatment also. A raised sleeping position for these patients is commonly recommended, but this is based on *common sense*, not evidence from RCTs. And strange enough, there is very little evidence of the advantages of pain medication in the symptomatic treatment of these children. Despite this, I'd like to argue that it would be irresponsible and unethical *not* to recommend pain medication.

CONCLUSION

In the words of Tonelli, '[C]linical medicine is, by its very nature, practical, prudential, and personal, and its practice more closely resembles casuistry than it does science.'[51] *Casuistry* here refers to case-based reasoning typical of law and ethics, where reasoning takes place primarily by analogy rather than deduction. The clinician compares the patient at hand with similar patients and pays attention to similarities and differences. Clinical research, of course, provides a source of potentially similar patients along with the challenge of determining whether they are 'similar enough'.[52]

Evidence from scientific studies is a necessary component of clinical decision making. Compared to the past, there is nowadays a lot more evidence, it is better than it once was, and it is easier to get one's hands on that evidence.[53]

Even scientific evidence is, however, a social product that is 'influenced by the variable power and authority held by different stakeholders (patients, medical researchers, hospital administrators, clinicians, policy makers etc.) in producing and determining the parameters for what counts as evidence'.[54]

Evidence from scientific studies reflects *general* knowledge, and the clinician has a *particular* patient in a *particular* situation. A good doctor is able to reflect on the evidence and apply it in the particular context.[55] A good doctor is aware of the values of the decision making: the values hidden in the evidence and the values hidden in the particular situation. He or she does not confuse personal opinion with evidence or personal ignorance with genuine scientific uncertainty.[56]

I wish to thank Dr Harri Hemilä for helpful discussions and several references.

REFERENCES

1 Galen. On the sects for beginners. In: Galen. *Three Treatises on the Nature of Science.* (Trans R. Walzer and M. Frede). Indianapolis, IN/Cambridge: Hackett Publishing Co; 1985 [2nd century]. p. 3.
2 Bernard C. *An Introduction to the Study of Experimental Medicine.* (Trans. HC Greene). New York, NY: Dover Publications; 1957 [1865]. pp. 206, 212.
3 Ford AC, Talley NJ, Spiegel BM, *et al.* Effect of fibre, antispasmodics, and peppermint oil in the treatment of irritable bowel syndrome: systematic review and meta-analysis. *BMJ.* 2008; 337: a2313.
4 Goodman J. *Ethics and Evidence-based Medicine.* Cambridge: Cambridge University Press; 2003.
5 Vandenbroucke JP. Evidence-based medicine and 'Médecine d'Observation'. *J Clin Epidemiol.* 1996; **49**: 1335–8.
6 Ibid.
7 Ashcroft R. Current epistemological problems in evidence-based medicine. In: ter Meulen R, Biller-Andorno N, Lenk C, Lie RK, editors. *Evidence-based Practice in Medicine and Health Care: a discussion of the ethical issues.* Berlin/Heidelberg/New York, NY: Springer; 2005. pp. 77–86.
8 Evidence-based medicine working group. Evidence-based medicine: a new approach to teaching the practice of medicine. *JAMA.* 1992; **268**: 2420–5.
9 Tonelli MR. The philosophical limits of evidence-based medicine. *Acad Med.* 1998; **73**: 1234–40.
10 Sackett DL, Rosenberg WMC, Gray JAM, *et al.* Evidence-based medicine: what it is and what it isn't. *BMJ.* 1996; **312**: 71–2.
11 Dutch Health Council, cited in: Vos R, Willems D, Houtepen R. Coordinating the norms and values of medical research, medical practice and patient worlds: the ethics of evidence-based medicine in 'boundary-fields' of medicine. In: ter Meulen R, Biller-Andorno N, Lenk C, *et al.*, editors. *Evidence-based Practice in Medicine and Health Care: a discussion of the ethical issues.* Berlin/Heidelberg/New York, NY: Springer; 2005.
12 Buetow S, Kenealy T. Evidence-based medicine: the need for a new definition. *J Eval Clin Pract.* 2000; **6**: 85–92.
13 Timmermans S, Mauck A. The promises and pitfalls of evidence-based medicine. *Health Affairs.* 2005; **24**: 18–28.
14 Tonelli MR, op. cit.
15 Feinstein AR, Horwitz RI. Problems in the 'evidence' of 'evidence-based medicine'. *Am J Med.* 1997; **103**: 529–35.
16 Vos R, Houtepen R, Horstman K. Evidence-based medicine and power shifts in health care systems. In: ter Meulen R, Biller-Andorno N, Lenk C, *et al.*, editors. *Evidence-based Practice in Medicine and Health Care: a discussion of the ethical issues.* Berlin/Heidelberg/New York, NY: Springer; 2005.

17 Evans M. Pictures of the patient: medicine, science and the humanities. In: Evans M, Sweeney K, editors. *The Human Side of Medicine*. London: Royal College of General Practitioners; 1998. Occasional Paper no. 76. pp. 1–16.
18 Tonelli MR, op. cit.
19 Charlton BG, Miles A. The rise and fall of EBM. *Q J Med*. 1998; **91**: 371–4.
20 Tonelli MR. Evidence-free medicine: forgoing evidence in clinical decision making. *Perspectives in Biology and Medicine*. 2009; **52**: 319–31.
21 Gerber A, Hentzelt F, Lauterbach KW. Can evidence-based medicine implicitly rely on current concepts of disease or does it have to develop its own definition? *Journal of Medical Ethics*. 2007; **33**: 394–9.
22 Kuhn T. *The Structure of Scientific Revolutions*. 2nd ed. Chicago: University of Chicago Press; 1970. p. 175.
23 Feinstein AR, Horwitz RI, op. cit.
24 Sackett DL, Richardson WS, Rosenberg W *et al*. *Evidence-based Medicine: how to practice and teach EBM*. London: Churchill Livingstone; 1997. p. 94.
25 Hill AB. Reflections on the controlled trial. *Ann Rheum Dis*. 1966; **25**: 107–13.
26 Liberati A, Vineis P. Defining a proper background for discussing evidence-based medicine. In: ter Meulen R, Biller-Andorno N, Lenk C, *et al.*, editors. *Evidence-based Practice in Medicine and Health Care: a discussion of the ethical issues*. Berlin/Heidelberg/New York, NY: Springer; 2005.
27 Feinstein AR, Horwitz RI, op. cit.
28 Greenhalgh T, Taylor R. How to read a paper: papers that go beyond numbers (qualitative research). *BMJ*. 1997; **315**: 740–3.
29 Green J, Britten N. Qualitative research and evidence based medicine. *BMJ*. 1998; **316**: 1230–2.
30 Rawlins M. *De testimonio*: on the evidence for decisions about the use of therapeutic interventions. *Lancet*. 2008; **372**: 2152–61.
31 Poynard T, Munteanu M, Ratziu V. Truth survival in clinical research: an evidence-based requiem? *Ann Intern Med*. 2002; **136**: 888–95.
32 Rawlins M, op. cit.
33 Houtepen R, Biller-Andorno N, Dickenson D, *et al*. Recommendations from the Evibase project. In: ter Meulen R, Biller-Andorno N, Lenk C, *et al.*, editors. *Evidence-based Practice in Medicine and Health Care: discussion of the ethical issues*. Berlin/Heidelberg/New York, NY: Springer; 2005.
34 Hardwig J. The role of trust in knowledge. *Journal of Philosophy*. 1991; **88**: 693–708.
35 Norman GR. Examining the assumptions of evidence-based medicine. *J Eval Clin Pract*. 1999; **5**: 139–47.
36 Feinstein AR, Horwitz RI, op. cit.
37 Goodman J, op. cit.
38 Parker M. Whither our art? Clinical wisdom and evidence-based medicine. *Medicine, Health Care and Philosophy*. 2002; **5**: 273–80.
39 Norman GR, op. cit.
40 Bagshaw SM, Bellomo R. The need to reform our assessment of evidence from clinical trials: a commentary. *Philosophy, Ethics, and Humanities in Medicine*. 2008; **3**: 23. doi:10.1186/1747-5341-3-23.
41 Charlton BG, Miles A, op. cit.

42 Goldenberg MJ. On evidence and evidence-based medicine: lessons from the philosophy of science. *Social Science & Medicine*. 2006; **62**: 2621–32.
43 Ibid.
44 Evans M, op. cit.
45 Tonelli MR 1998, op. cit.
46 Nummenmaa J. Näyttöön perustuvat hoitosuositukset ja yleislääkärin työ [*Evidence-based Guidelines and General Practice*] [dissertation]. Tampere: Acta Universitatis Tamperensis [University of Tampere] 1204; 2007 (in Finnish).
47 Goodman J, op. cit.
48 Molewijk AC, Stiggelbout AM, Otten W, *et al*. Implicit normativity in evidence-based medicine: a plea for integrated empirical ethics research. *Health Care Anal*. 2003; **11**: 69–92.
49 Ibid.
50 Louhiala P. Medicine as a moral enterprise. In: Evans M, Louhiala P, Puustinen R. editors. *Philosophy for Medicine: applications in a clinical context*. Oxford: Radcliffe Medical Press; 2004. pp. 135–42.
51 Tonelli MR 1998, op. cit.
52 Ibid.
53 Goodman J, op. cit.
54 Goldenberg MJ, op. cit.
55 Saunders J. The practice of clinical medicine as an art and as a science. *J Med Ethics: Medical Humanities*. 2000; **26**: 18–22.
56 Ibid.

5

Paternalism, power and autonomy

IONA HEATH

PLAYING GOD

At their paternalistic worst, doctors are accused of 'playing God'. This suggests continuing relevance for the primordial myth of the loss of paradise and its exposition of the fundamental tension between paternalism and autonomy.

> And the Lord God formed man of the dust of the ground, and breathed into his nostrils the breath of life; and man became a living soul.
> And the Lord God planted a garden eastward in Eden; and there he put the man whom he had formed.
> And out of the ground made the Lord God to grow every tree that is pleasant to the sight, and good for food; the tree of life also in the midst of the garden, and the tree of knowledge of good and evil.[1]
>
> And the Lord God took the man, and put him into the garden of Eden to dress it and to keep it.
> And the Lord God commanded the man, saying, Of every tree of the garden thou mayest freely eat:
> but of the tree of the knowledge of good and evil, thou shalt not eat of it: for in the day that thou eatest thereof thou shalt surely die.[2]
>
> Now the serpent was more subtil than any beast of the field which the Lord God had made. And he said unto the woman, Yea, hath God said, Ye shall not eat of every tree of the garden?

> And the woman said unto the serpent, We may eat of the fruit of the trees of the garden:
> but of the fruit of the tree which is in the midst of the garden, God hath said, Ye shall not eat of it, neither shall ye touch it, lest ye die.
> And the serpent said unto the woman, Ye shall not surely die:
> for God doth know that in the day ye eat thereof, then your eyes shall be opened, and ye shall be as gods, knowing good and evil.
> And when the woman saw that the tree was good for food, and that it was pleasant to the eyes, and a tree to be desired to make one wise, she took of the fruit thereof, and did eat, and gave also unto her husband with her; and he did eat.[3]

Eleven verses later, we find God's response:

> And unto Adam he said, Because thou hast hearkened unto the voice of thy wife, and hast eaten of the tree, of which I commanded thee, saying, Thou shalt not eat of it: cursed is the ground for thy sake; in sorrow shalt thou eat of it all the days of thy life;
> thorns also and thistles shall it bring forth to thee; and thou shalt eat the herb of the field:
> in the sweat of thy face shalt thou eat bread, till thou return unto the ground; for out of it wast thou taken: for dust thou art, and unto dust shalt thou return.[4]

> And the Lord God said, Behold, the man is become as one of us, to know good and evil: and now, lest he put forth his hand, and take also of the tree of life, and eat, and live for ever:
> therefore the Lord God sent him forth from the garden of Eden, to till the ground from whence he was taken.[5]

The subtlety of this ancient poetic narrative contrasts very starkly with the contemporary enthusiasm for portraying medical paternalism as bad and patient autonomy as good. The story of the expulsion from paradise makes it very clear that the relationship between paternalism and autonomy is profoundly ambiguous and that both are compounded of goods and harms.

Ambiguity

Gods protect, but they also punish. In his poem, 'The Last Pain', William Empson alludes to the ambiguity at the heart of the human relationship with the paternalism of the gods:

> Ambiguous gifts, as what gods give must be.[6]

When doctors 'play god', the relationship is no less ambiguous and concerns:

> the shades of grey between the doctor's duty to respect autonomy on the one hand, and to act beneficently on the other.[7]

The story of the Garden of Eden demonstrates that paternalism protects people from the realities of the world and the imminence of death at the cost of a naïve innocence; autonomy confers self-determination but this is always accompanied by responsibility for one's own actions and an inevitable sense of guilt when things go wrong. Within contemporary society, knowledge seems to be seen as a constituent of happiness, whereas knowledge is always of both good and evil and so can and does actively undermine happiness. Human knowledge is most fundamentally of the finitude of life and is forever accompanied by the fear of death.

In *Paradise Lost,* John Milton accepts that there are limits to the extent of knowledge of pain and suffering that a human mind can tolerate.

> But knowledge is as food, and needs no less
> Her temperance over Appetite, to know
> In measure what the mind may well contain.[8]

It is possible that a beneficent paternalism can provide a measure of protection from the destructive effect of an excess of knowledge.

'Presentism' and the history of medical paternalism

In a recent article, Laurence B McCullough describes the founding story of bioethics within which medical paternalism was an accepted ethical norm in the history of Western medical ethics and was widespread in clinical practice until bioethics came along to correct this grave wrong by creating a shift in the ethical norms and practice of medicine.[9] McCullough analyses the writings of John Gregory (1724–73) and Thomas Percival (1740–1804) in order to demonstrate that the relationship between medical paternalism and patient autonomy has always been a complex and challenging one and that the oppositional rhetoric within contemporary bioethics represents a damaging simplification. Further, the distortions of the founding story serve, in effect, to deprofessionalise bioethics and to undermine the fiduciary relationship of doctors to their patients and the protections this relationship offers.

There is almost always a balance to be struck between paternalism and autonomy within the therapeutic relationship between patient and doctor, while recognising that both parties need some measure of power, agency and autonomy.[10] This balance is subject to many tensions, mediated by the degree to which patient autonomy is overwhelmed by the severity of illness or by fear; the limits of information in promoting autonomy; the extent to which autonomy can be bolstered by social relationships and by the balance of power and trust within the relationship between doctor and patient; the degree to which the rhetoric of choice has become a substitute for autonomy; issues of futility towards the end of life; the balance between individual autonomy and societal aspirations to improve population health; and the relationship between the autonomy of patients and the clinical autonomy of doctors. I will explore each of these in turn: ultimately, as in *Genesis*, the fundamental tension remains that between knowledge and fear.

Autonomy versus heteronomy

It is too easy to assume that the most serious threat to the autonomy of patients comes from the attitudes and paternalistic arrogance of doctors. The most fundamental threat often derives directly from the heteronomy of the body. Heteronomy is the opposite of autonomy and implies subjection to an external law. The paradox is that the human spirit feels itself to be free and autonomous and yet it remains always subject to the heteronomy of the body. Sickness in the body limits its capacities and thereby compromises the autonomy of the person to an extent that varies from the barely perceptible to the utterly devastating.

> They form a strange pair: the free spirit celebrated by modern philosophy and the deterministic body known by modern science. But a pair they are.[11]

When Jake gets the hot, cramping pain in his abdomen, all he can think about is the imminence of diarrhoea, and his pressing need for a toilet. His dignity and autonomy are sabotaged by the frailty of his body. To a lesser extent, Liz's autonomy is compromised by her embarrassment over the intimate nature of her health problem. Thus, in many situations, the greatest threat to the autonomy of patients is not the paternalism of doctors, but the compromises that are imposed by the illness itself.

Both patient and doctor have power and agency and these are by no means necessarily opposed to each other. The purpose of the therapeutic consultation is to combine and so augment the agency of both parties in the interests of enabling the patient to regain balance and self-determination in the face of illness and suffering. The consultation always has the potential to be a meeting of experts[12] – the doctor being the expert in medical science and the patient being the expert in his or her own values, biography and social context. Little insists that:

> It is not productive to see power solely as domination.[13]

Much of the rhetoric, which portrays medical paternalism as bad and patient autonomy as an unequivocal good, seems to interpret the distribution of power within the doctor–patient relationship as being a zero sum. Anything that increases the doctor's power is seen to necessarily reduce that of the patient and vice versa. However, human relationships always have the potential to augment the power of both parties. Facing the challenges of illness and suffering brought on by the inevitable heteronomy of the body, both patients and doctors have the capacity to combine and so enhance their separate powers.[14]

Fear

Rachel's mother is clearly disempowered by her fears for her daughter, and she is living the connection between responsibility and guilt that is inherent in autonomous adulthood. Both Liz and Jen are impeded by their fears of the implications of their diagnoses. Geoff has withdrawn into himself, possibly as a means of coping with overwhelming fears of his complete loss of independence and the destruction of his previous capacity for life. Returning to Milton, he has perhaps been offered more knowledge of his bleak future than his mind can 'well contain'. In a sense, Jane is making a futile attempt to shelter Jen from the fruit of the tree of knowledge which is the immediacy of death.

Different individuals find it more or less easy to exert or even recognise their capacity for autonomy. Family and cultural traditions make it more or less acceptable to 'make a fuss', and Jen seems to find it almost impossible to actively ask for help, either personal or professional. Indeed, one wonders to what extent she has been genuinely involved in the decisions about her chemotherapy. Social structures can actively impede or promote an individual's capacity for autonomy. Poverty, lack of education, lack of language skills and/or low self-esteem may make it difficult to exert autonomy, which may be compromised differently for different individuals within different societal and cultural contexts.

The limits of information

Knowledge and information help to promote the autonomy and agency of patients. Rachel's ability to cope is enhanced by the information that is provided by her specialist nurse, Dax, and perhaps even more by the solidarity shown by her friend Leroy and the information that he is able to find for her on the Internet. Jen would have been helped to preserve her dignity if she had been warned and prepared for the sudden onset of severe diarrhoea. Her autonomy was directly compromised by a lack of crucial information. However, the experiences of sick healthcare professionals suggests that knowledge and information only go so far and can be all too easily undermined by the effects of fear, which saps autonomy and paralyses the exercise of choice. The challenge for the doctor is to provide information without exacerbating fear.

Social relationships: myth and belonging

Once autonomy is damaged, it is not easy to restore, and in his account of the story of Philoctetes, Sophocles (wonderfully interpreted by Seamus

Heaney) explores his understanding of social connections as the beginning of re-establishing self-confidence and self-determination. The restoration of individual autonomy is a social not an individual endeavour. Philoctetes was left stranded by Odysseus on the way to Troy because of a festering wound on his foot that exuded an unbearable stench.

> I am the one
> That dumped him, him and his cankered foot –
> Or what had been a foot before it rotted
> And ate itself with ulcers.
> It was awful.[15]

Alone on the island of Lemnos for 10 years, Philoctetes became increasingly angered and embittered.

> Festering inside and out.
> Contrary, hard and proud.[16]

Eventually the Greeks return once they understand that they cannot defeat the Trojans without Philoctetes' bow and arrows, which he has inherited from the great hero, Heracles, half-man and half-god. On this occasion, Odysseus is accompanied by the young Neoptolemus, the son of the now-dead Achilles. Odysseus wants to use Neoptolemus to trick Philoctetes into giving up his weapons, but Neoptolemus is overwhelmed by pity for his predicament and sees the importance of human contact to healing the often self-inflicted isolation of the sick.

> There's a whole economy of kindness
> Possible in the world; befriend a friend
> And the chance of it's increased and multiplied.[17]

Carol's attempts to reach Jake show how difficult it can be to break down the barriers and Geoff appears to be resigned to solitude as the most preferable of his very limited options so that only Jen is able to maintain the most tenuous of connections with him.

The relationships between patients and doctors, and other health professionals, such as Rachel's Dax, can be a very important part of re-establishing the all-important social contact, provided that the clinician, unlike Liz's Dr Patience, is prepared to offer an authentic human relationship rather than one that is merely technical and/or hierarchical.

> If, therefore, we as general practitioners are to make our unique contribution ..., it will be as personal doctors whose way of listening, examining, diagnosing,

> advising, treating and monitoring has as its objective not only the cure or control of disease but the protection or expansion of our patients' stature, autonomy and personal space. That is the kind of health we can deliver, even to people with disease, even to people who are dying. We do it in the consultation.[18]

Trust

Some degree of trust is essential to social relationships, which is why Neoptolemus has to work so hard to overcome Philoctetes' deep distrust of Odysseus. Trust is essential to the establishing of relationships between human beings, and the fiduciary relationship between patient and doctor necessitates additional dimensions of trust. The patient must feel able to trust that the doctor has the necessary and appropriate training and skill, and that he or she is functioning within an ethical framework that prioritises the needs of the patient above those of the doctor. The autonomy of the sick is fragile and is all too easily undermined by a failure of trust, and in today's increasingly commercialised healthcare context, trust may be rapidly eroded if the patient perceives the doctor to have a conflict of interest or if they begin to understand that the doctor's own autonomy is being eroded by, for example, resource constraints or political or bureaucratic coercion. The sister on Geoff's ward is almost certainly under pressure to discharge patients as early as possible.

Onora O'Neill brings us back to *Genesis*, noting that breaches of trust date back to the Garden of Eden and that trust is always, in the end, a gamble.

> [T]rust is needed precisely because all guarantees are incomplete. Since trust has to be placed without guarantees, it is inevitably sometimes misplaced: others let us down and we let others down. When this happens trust and relationships based on trust are both damaged. Trust, it is constantly observed, is hard earned and easily dissipated. It is valuable social capital and not to be squandered.[19]

Almost all doctors have direct experience of having done something that resulted in the loss of the hard-earned trust of a patient. Doctors know just how easily trust is dissipated and so are often peculiarly sensitive to changes to the context of healthcare that seem to threaten trust. O'Neill herself draws attention to the vogue for ever-heightened accountability, which, she asserts, does little to promote trust but that superimposes 'managerial targets on bureaucratic process, burdening and even paralysing many of those who have to comply'.

In the end, as Sophocles so clearly understood, trust is a product of the quality of the relationship between people so that it is able to withstand the inevitable failures of both parties. Forgiveness can only be both offered and accepted within relationships that are characterised by trust. Patients who perceive that their doctors do not listen to them or do not, in some sense, even see them, are unlikely to find those doctors particularly trustworthy. The reverse also holds.

Authenticity

In order to constitute social connectedness and to provide a basis for trust, the relationship between patient and healthcare professional has to be between two human subjects,[20] with both parties fully present. Significantly, presence is the fifth component of Little's fivefold root of an ethics of surgery, described as both a virtue and a duty.

The nursing sister on Geoff's ward does not even attempt to see Jen as a human subject and completely fails to imagine her predicament. In an important sense, the nurse is absent and so unable to 'see' the patient.

This failure of recognition seems to lie at the root of stereotypical medical arrogance and paternalism. The doctor focuses on the disease rather than the patient:

> [T]he prevailing commitment to accurate diagnosis of disease – which is the hallmark of the modern physician – turns on the notion that there is a pure disease state which is, ideally, distinct from the patient. Thus, the patient is seen as a kind of 'translucent screen' on which the disease is projected. In consequence, … the patient's subjective experiencing of illness is ignored in favor of an objective, quantitative account of a disease state.[21]

The doctor sees the map of medical science rather than the territory of the patient's subjective suffering. Presence is much more than the merely physical, although this is clearly a basic prerequisite. Beyond the physical is the commitment to bring the necessary resources of curiosity, imagination and kindness, alongside the courage to look the patient in the eye and to acknowledge the shared experience of human frailty and finitude. Authenticity and presence demand moral effort.

Over recent years, doctors have worked hard to refocus on the individual person who has become the patient, but there is a danger that this achievement is now being actively undermined as computer-prompted, disease-focused targets, re-emphasise the disease, again at the expense of the person of the patient.

There is a clear and increasing tension between the enthusiasm of public health medicine to achieve targets and the autonomy of individual patients; between the inevitable utilitarianism of the political and societal perspective and the clinician's imperative to prioritise the needs of individual patients. The public health approach is based on a normative view of health that ignores the multiplicity of ways in which individuals develop their own concepts of what it means to be healthy that make sense in the context of their own particular values, opportunities and family and social context.

> Although health is naturally the goal of the doctor's activity, it is not actually 'made' by the doctor. Connected to this is something further: the goal of health is not a condition that is clearly definable from within the medical art. For illness is a social state of affairs. It is also a psychological-moral state of affairs, much more than a fact that is determinable from within the natural sciences.[22]

A public health discourse treats a normative definition of health as an end itself whereas individuals are more likely to see their own health as a means to other ends of their own devising.

Discussions of patient 'compliance' with treatment make these tensions explicit, and the terminology seems in itself to reject the possibility that the patient, and the patient alone, has the right to decide whether or not he or she will take a prescribed drug. What is needed is a term that makes explicit the likelihood of divergence between the aspirations of medical science and those of individual patients striving to make the best of complicated and challenging lives: indeed, the usefulness of disagreement as the basis of dialectic within a meeting of experts. If the dignity and autonomy of each patient is to be genuinely respected, the outcome of the consultation will often conflict with recommended medical guidance. Fundamentally, this is simply another manifestation of that familiar conflict between the utilitarian benefit of the many and the dignity and freedom of the individual, which has persisted throughout history as each successive utopian dream has degenerated into tyranny. The dream of perfect health is the contemporary utopia and comes, as always, accompanied by coercion.[23] Medical paternalism is rendered inevitable if health services are committed to a normative view of health and if doctors are expected to play a role as agents of distributive social justice.

The essential feature of a genuine dialogue between parties, both of whom have power and autonomy, including that between doctor and patient, is that neither party controls the interaction and both can be changed by it.

> A patient-professional encounter is a discourse; a dialogue is an interpersonal mode of being which at its best may be called authentic interaction. The 'magic' of authentic interaction is that we do not completely control it as individuals, but are caught up in it and give in to its own movement.[24]

This is the very opposite of an encounter whose purpose is to achieve compliance.

Choice

If a doctor or other clinician perceives his or her role simply as a purveyor of information, he or she has no capacity for change and there is no real exchange. Worries about medical paternalism have meant that young doctors may now be taught, some times and in some places, to provide information to patients and to offer them choices but to avoid advice as to which course of action might be preferable.

> Autonomy implies the right to make mistakes, to have regrets, to choose unwisely, to behave foolishly.[25]

Yet, some of the treatment choices that patients are asked to make are almost horrifyingly serious and can have very far-reaching consequences. Is it fair to expect patients to shoulder the responsibility for these choices entirely alone, especially when their autonomy is already compromised by anxiety, pain or sickness?

> ... the instinctive resistance practising physicians often have towards overemphasizing autonomy in the doctor-patient relationship. One cannot abandon persons to their autonomy when they are in difficult straits.[26]

To an important extent, health is a prerequisite just as much as a consequence of choice.[27] Annemarie Mol contrasts the logic of choice with that of care:

> The logic of choice is concerned with individuals who wish to be free. The individuals who figure in the logic of care would die if they were left alone. They owe their very ability to act to others.[28]

Patients often ask, 'What would you do doctor?' or 'What would you want for *your* mother?' In some places, young doctors are now advised to resist such questions, but to do so is to refuse a relationship between human subjects. Patients know very well that a doctor would never refuse to answer such a question if it was posed by his or her own mother in the context of an authentic relationship. Clearly, a patient should never be told what the doctor would do in similar circumstances without careful caveats about the personal nature of such decisions and about alternative decisions being equally valid and appropriate for different people, but, in a sense, the doctor's taking of a position can open up the field of decision making and make the alternatives clearer so that decisions become easier. Further, the doctor offers to share at least some of the responsibility for a decision, the consequences of which could be devastating. Abandoning a patient to a difficult choice of treatment options, however much supporting information is provided can paralyse decision making through fear. Equally, doctors prepared to share the responsibility for the outcome of a difficult decision put themselves in a position to share the burden of guilt if things go wrong. Part of the intention is to offer social connection and to help the patient, like Philoctetes, feel less isolated and alone.

Futility

Particularly in terminal illness, patients may demand treatments that their doctors believe to be not only distressing but futile. Is it paternalistic or immoral to refuse such treatments?

> Patients do not have a right to useless treatments nor doctors a duty to provide them on demand. Autonomy is not enhanced or respected where one choice offers no reasonable prospect of a particular outcome.[29]

In his book about the last illness of his mother, Susan Sontag, David Rieff describes her ruthless desperation to remain alive and her willingness to undergo any treatment to this end, however small the chances of success.[30] The story illustrates what happens when anything short of the technically possible is regarded as rationing, and her son asks why no one was prepared to protect her through the exercise of humane clinical judgement. Yet, conversely, within a publicly funded healthcare system such as the National Health Service (the NHS) in the United Kingdom, funding constraints may limit the range of treatment choice available for patients so that issues of social solidarity and justice impede individual autonomy. The hidden benefit can sometimes be the restraint of excessive and harmful medical enthusiasm. Neither power nor autonomy is ever absolute.

Clinical autonomy

To a very real extent, the autonomy of patients is dependent on the autonomy of their doctors, and so it becomes important to examine the ways in which clinical autonomy can be impaired.[31] Perhaps most crucially, clinical power and autonomy is undermined by inadequate medical and technical knowledge and/or limited clinical skills. This in turn can be exacerbated by limited access to the essential support of colleagues with different and complementary expertise and by resource constraints that make it difficult or even impossible to gain access to investigations and treatment in a timely fashion. More recently, payment-for-performance systems have eroded clinical autonomy through systems of bureaucratic surveillance compounded by political coercion and financial incentives. With so much of the agenda of consultations now dictated from outside the conversation between patient and doctor within what Glyn Elwyn has described as the 'multivocal postmodern consultation',[32] it can be very easy for the priorities of the patient to be marginalised.

Beyond the technical

The goal of medical treatment is the restoration of a sense of wholeness so that the sick body no longer impedes the aspirations of the self. Technical expertise is essential but not sufficient and doctors also have a responsibility to try to augment the patient's capacity for 'mending through meaning'.[33] This involves purposeful dialogue between doctor and patient with the aim of discovering a coherent explanation of illness that makes sense to the sufferer and, by reducing fear, uncertainty and confusion, and by making room for optimism, boosts the body's innate capacity for mending.

It is known that meaning attached to the colour[34] or form of medication, the reputation of medicines resulting from advertising[35] or other forms of publicity, the relationship between the patient and the physician,[36] the attitude of the physician to the patient, and the degree to which the physician believes in the efficacy of the treatment can all have a measurable effect on the outcome of any given treatment.[37] For generations, doctors have deliberately cultivated ongoing relationships with their patients, based on an intentional positive regard for each patient, knowing intuitively and from experience that relationships that both patient and doctor enjoy produce better health outcomes for patients.[38]

Trends that minimise the importance of the subjectivity of both doctor and patient within conventional medicine appear to be driving patients to seek therapeutic relationships with alternative practitioners: there has been an explosion in demand for such care, leading to pressure for such alternatives to be publicly funded within national health services. As a result, technological and inter-subjective therapeutic power becomes divided between different roles instead of being combined and maximised so that the inter-subjective can be used systematically in order to maximise the effectiveness of scientific technologies of proven benefit.

The irony is that the current profligate destruction of the therapeutic capacity of doctors is occurring just as science itself may be beginning to explain the mechanism of those aspects of medical practice that have come to be regarded as unscientific and therefore redundant. As psychoneuroimmunology gradually unpicks the extraordinarily intricate interactions between the immune system, the autonomic nervous system and the subjective experience of the individual, the more we begin to understand the power of both positive and negative psychological states in promoting or undermining the healthy functioning of the human body.[39] It seems that supportive personal relationships, including, one must presume, relationships between doctors and patients, can diminish negative emotions and promote health through a positive impact on immune function.[40] This new linking of science and humanism looks likely to offer both new insights and new challenges to our notions of what it means to be human.

Knowledge and fear

People in receipt of healthcare and medical treatment need information and knowledge about their condition and, whenever they have the capacity, they can also be helped to retrieve and maximise their status as self-directed, morally autonomous individuals. However, as in the Garden of Eden and throughout all subsequent history, the fruit of the tree of knowledge is of good and evil and of the finitude of life, and this knowledge is forever accompanied by fear and suffering:

> Making all thought impossible but how
> And where and when I shall myself die.[41]

Doctors and other healthcare professionals have an ongoing responsibility to share the burdens of responsibility and fear, because whenever these burdens are laid aside, which, as our stories show, is done all too easily, care and treatment may become insensitive, unkind and even, on occasions, cruel.

REFERENCES

1 *Holy Bible, King James version,* Genesis, Chapter 2, verses 7–9.
2 *Holy Bible, King James version,* Genesis, Chapter 2, verses 15–17.
3 *Holy Bible, King James version,* Genesis, Chapter 3, verses 1–6.
4 *Holy Bible, King James version,* Genesis, Chapter 3, verses 17–19.
5 *Holy Bible, King James version,* Genesis, Chapter 3, verses 22–3.
6 Quoted in Ricks C. *The Force Of Poetry.* Oxford: Oxford University Press; 1984.
7 Bewley S, Friend J, Mezey G. *Violence Against Women.* London: RCOG Press; 1997.
8 Milton J. *Paradise Lost* vii: 126–8.
9 McCullough LB. Was bioethics founded on historical and conceptual mistakes about medical paternalism? *Bioethics.* 2011; **25**(2): 66–74.
10 Popper K. *Conjectures and Refutations.* Abingdon: Routledge Classics; 2002 [1963]. p. 497.
11 Mol A. *The Logic Of Care: health and the problem of patient choice.* Abingdon: Routledge; 2006. p. 43.
12 Tuckett D, Boulton M, Olson C, *et al. Meetings Between Experts: an approach to sharing ideas in medical consultations.* London: Tavistock; 1985.
13 Little M. The fivefold root of an ethics of surgery. *Bioethics.* 2002; **16**(3): 183–201.
14 Foucault M. *Power/Knowledge: selected interviews and other writings 1972–1977.* London: Harvester Press; 1980.
15 Heaney S. *The Cure At Troy.* Derry: Field Day; 1990. p. 3.
16 Heaney S. *The Cure At Troy.* Derry: Field Day; 1990. p. 13.
17 Heaney S. *The Cure At Troy.* Derry: Field Day; 1990. p. 37.
18 Metcalfe D. The crucible. *J Roy Coll Gen Pract.* 1986; **36**: 349–54.
19 O'Neill O. *The Philosophy of Trust.* BBC Reith Lectures; 2002. Available at: www.bbc.co.uk/radio4/reith2002/lecture1.shtml.
20 Nessa J. *Talk As Medical Work: discourse analysis of patient–doctor communication in general practice.* Bergen: University of Bergen; 1999.
21 Toombs SK. *The Meaning Of Illness.* Dordrecht: Kluwer Academic Publishers; 1993.
22 Gadamer H-G. *The Enigma Of Health: the art of healing in a scientific age.* Stanford: Stanford University Press; 1996.
23 Heath I. A wolf in sheep's clothing: a critical look at the ethics of drug taking. *BMJ.* 2003; **327**: 856–8.

24 Nessa J, Malterud K. Tell me what is wrong with me: a discourse analysis approach to the concept of patient autonomy. *Journal of Medical Ethics*. 1998; **24**: 394–400.
25 Skrabanek P. *The Death Of Humane Medicine*. London: The Social Affairs Unit; 1994.
26 Thomasma DC. Establishing the moral basis of medicine: Edmund D Pellegrino's philosophy of medicine. *J Med Philosophy*. 1990; **15**: 245–67.
27 Roberts MJ, Reich MR. Ethical analysis in public health. *Lancet*. 2002; **359**: 1055–9.
28 Mol A. *The Logic Of Care: health and the problem of patient choice*. Abingdon: Routledge; 2006. p. 72.
29 Saunders J. Perspectives on CPR: resuscitation or resurrection? *Clin Med JRCPL*. 2001; **1**: 457–60.
30 Rieff D. *Swimming In a Sea Of Death: a son's memoir*. London: Granta; 2008.
31 Williamson C. Alford's theoretical political framework and its application to interests in health care now. *Br J Gen Pract*. 2008; **58(552)**: 512–16.
32 Elwyn G. Arriving at the postmodern medical consultation. *Primary Care*. 2005; **5**: 287–91.
33 Moerman, D. Physiology and symbols: the anthropological implications of the placebo effect. In: Romanucci-Ross L, Moerman,DE, Tancredi LR, editors. *The Anthropology Of Medicine: from culture to method*. Westport: Bergin and Garvey; 1997.
34 de Craen AJ, Roos PJ, Leonard de Vries, *et al*. Effect of colour of drugs: systematic review of perceived effect of drugs and of their effectiveness. *BMJ*. 1996; **313**: 1624–6.
35 Branthwaite A, Cooper P. Analgesic effects of branding in treatment of headaches. *BMJ*. 1981; **282**: 1576–8.
36 Ekeland, T.-J. The healing context and efficacy in psychotherapy: psychotherapy and the placebo phenomenon. *International Journal of Psychotherapy*. 1997; **2**: 77–87.
37 Di Blasi Z, Harkness E, Ernst E, *et al*. Influence of context effects on health outcomes: a systematic review. *Lancet*. 2001; **357**: 757–62.
38 Krupnick JL, Sotsky SM, Simmens S, *et al*. The role of the therapeutic alliance in psychotherapy and pharmacotherapy outcome: findings in the National Institute of Mental Health Treatment of Depression Collaborative Research Program. *J Consult Clin Psychol*. 1996; **64**: 532–9.
39 Fleshner M, Laudenslager ML. Psychoneuroimmunology: then and now. *Behavioral & Cognitive Neuroscience Reviews*. 2004; **3**: 114–30.
40 Kiecolt-Glaser JK, McGuire L, Robles TF, *et al*. Emotions, morbidity, and mortality: new perspectives from psychoneuroimmunology. *Annual Review of Psychology*. 2002; **53**: 83–107.
41 Larkin P. Aubade. In: *Collected Poems*. London: Faber and Faber; 1988. p. 208.

CHAPTER 6

Symptoms without disease: territory without a map

JILL GORDON

Nobody wants an anonymous illness.[1]

In the novel *Regeneration*[2] Pat Barker describes one of the techniques used during the Great War to treat soldiers with hysterical mutism:

> The patient had been strapped to a chair for periods of twenty minutes at a time, and very strong electric current applied to his neck and throat. Hot plates had been applied repeatedly to the back of the throat, and lighted cigarettes to the tongue.[2]

This is no exaggeration for the sake of dramatic fiction. Barker's account is taken directly from a monograph by Lewis R Yealland, the Canadian neurologist who pioneered the use of electricity and other physical treatments for shell-shocked soldiers at the National Hospital in London.[3] Pat Barker recreates one of the treatment episodes exactly as described by Yealland, with just one alteration: in Barker's novel, the scene is viewed through the eyes of psychiatrist WHR Rivers. Rivers watches as Yealland applies electric shocks to the young soldier's mouth, throat and neck until he is forced to speak, so that Yealland can declare triumphantly that he has been cured. Rivers's treatment approach is diametrically opposed to Yealland's. He is pioneering new methods of treating shell shock by showing gentle, even fatherly, kindness to the soldiers while they work their own way through the trauma that they have suffered – the nightmares, flashbacks and intrusive thoughts that we now accept as the *sine qua non* of post-traumatic stress disorder (PTSD).

One of Rivers's patients was the poet Siegfried Sassoon. In *Sherston's Progress* Sassoon wrote:

> Shell-shock. How many a brief bombardment had its long-delayed after-effect in the minds of these survivors, many of whom had looked at their companions and laughed while the inferno did its best to destroy them. Not then was their evil hour, but now; now, in the sweating, suffocation of nightmare, in paralysis of limbs, in the stammering of dislocated speech. Worst of all, in the disintegration of those qualities through which they had been so gallant and selfless and uncomplaining – this, in the finer types of men, was the unspeakable tragedy of shell shock.[4]

Shell shock has now been renamed post-traumatic stress disorder (PTSD). It occurs when humans face horrors that are so overwhelming that any normal person could be expected to succumb – a physical assault, a severe motor vehicle accident, a rape, an armed hold-up – I have seen each of these traumatic events trigger PTSD in strong, resourceful people who have been pushed beyond their emotional limits. The condition was not well understood at the time of the Great War and treatment was based on the mistaken belief that the nervous system could be 'shocked' by shelling in a way that was essentially physical. It was some time before the mechanism of PTSD was sufficiently well understood as to guide treatment.

In Chapter 2 of this volume, Martyn Evans defines treatment as 'ordinarily an intelligent, purposive, intentional and interpersonal activity'. In medicine, treatment maps are constructed by collaborations, sometimes over many centuries, in which an increased understanding of disease mechanisms leads towards a cure or cures. In about 1500 BCE the Egyptians knew at least three things about diabetes – that it created sweet-tasting urine, that it caused wasting and that it was fatal. They made the first marks on the 'map' for its diagnosis and management, but it was not until the mid-19th century that malfunction of the pancreas was identified as the root cause of diabetes and was seen to be a starting point for treatment. Even then, it was not until 1922 that a patient undertook a successful journey out of illness territory when given insulin. Since that time, many lives have been saved and many more details have been added to the diabetes treatment map. These developments have improved the chances of a normal life span for children like Rachel, and the map is now so clear that we can say with certainty that Nahkira Harris, whose case is described in Chapter 8, should not have died.

Jen's cancer, by contrast, can be represented by a treatment map with many paths – chemotherapy, radiotherapy, surgery, palliative care – a reflection of the fact that a single specific way of targeting the disease, based on fundamental biological research, has not been found. There is always a possibility that the cancer map will be radically redrawn in the coming years, just as the map for gastric cancer has been redrawn by the discovery of a specific cause in *helicobacter pylori* (*H. pylori*) infection.

The map for Jake's irritable bowel syndrome (IBS) is an even less complete treatment map and is one that is complicated by the conceptual divide between 'mental' and 'physical' illnesses. This is the point at which we begin to talk about symptoms without disease, or 'territory without a map'. It is this conceptual divide that made possible the construction of two distinctly different treatment maps for shell shock, one of which we would regard today as tantamount to torture, the other as mainstream. Doctors like Yealland and Rivers operated with remarkable autonomy, and their approaches were as much a reflection of their own worldviews as of the problem that they were trying to solve. Yealland, like Mesmer (*see* Chapter 9) was bold and self-confident. He was willing to put his responsibilities to the suffering individual behind his determination to succeed in returning soldiers to the Front. He was willing to put expediency before compassion. In *The Common Sense Of Science* Jacob Bronowski argues that neither the boldness of men like Yealland nor even the appearance of success is a valid criterion for good science:

> We are faced every day with actions of which our own code of conduct makes us ashamed, but which we find compelling if we are to battle with the hard facts of society.... Beyond all our actions stands the larger shadow: how are we to choose between what we have been taught to think right and something else which manifestly succeeds?[5]

For Bronowski, scientific and moral integrity are inseparable; success cannot be said to have occurred if it is success in only one of the two domains. Yealland may have succeeded in returning soldiers to the Front by shaming and blaming them, but his 'treatment' was often followed by the manifestation of different hysterical symptoms and, in other cases, it probably resulted in young men who had lost all hope dying on the battlefield. 'Manifest success' that runs counter to human values seems ultimately to find ways of undoing itself.

Another story connected to the treatment of shell shock was made into a film: *The King's Speech*.[6] Colin Firth plays the part of the Duke of York (later King George VI) who must overcome a stammer in order to deliver speeches to his subjects. Like Yealland and Rivers, speech therapist Lionel Logue experiments with all manner of 'treatments' in which he sincerely believes, but for which there is little if any evidence. The treatments include rolling around on the floor and swearing. They also include treatments for which evidence has subsequently emerged, such as singing and reducing auditory feedback. More than anything, however, the treatment has one important similarity with the treatment used by Rivers – both men, one wittingly and one perhaps unwittingly, were able to create a therapeutic relationship. Lionel Logue lacks formal qualifications in speech therapy, but he has experience in treating young men who returned from the Great War with disordered speech. He approaches his clients with what Carl Rogers called unconditional positive regard. The Duke of York finds in Lionel a friend for the first time in his life, and he responds to the encouragement, in the literal sense of the word, with a growing sense of self-confidence.

The film takes the usual liberties with the true story on which it is based, but it is a fact that Lionel Logue and King George VI remained friends for the rest of their lives.

The stories recounted in *Regeneration* and *The King's Speech* pose questions about the nature of therapy when an illness has no accompanying evidence of physical pathology that we can detect with present-day tools – when the map is largely blank.

The patients in our stories – Rachel, Liz, Jake, Geoff and Jen, have experienced physical pathology – diabetes, cervical pathology, epilepsy, psoriasis, a stroke and cancer. However, they also have the usual emotional responses: fear, uncertainty, helplessness and grief. Not only does it appear arguable that anxiety and depression are part and parcel of serious illness, but patients like Jake can also present with what is often called a functional disorder – in Jake's case, his bowel functions abnormally, but there is no obvious pathology there.

Reflecting on the ways in which Rivers and Logue treated symptoms without evidence of disease raises some general questions about treatment – for example: Is it a moral requirement for a therapist to hold a sincere belief in the efficacy of a particular treatment that s/he employs? To what extent should a treating doctor try to convey confidence in an unproven treatment? Does it matter *how* a treatment works, provided that it does? And is there any real difference between faith in unproven treatments and, say, religious faith?

The question of the therapist's beliefs poses a challenge in situations where the efficacy of a particular treatment cannot be easily assessed. In Western medical circles, the consensus would appear to be that patients have the right to know whether a treatment has been fully validated. This is not quite so difficult in circumstances where new treatments must be tried in order to make progress – for example, in the treatment of certain cancers. However, in this chapter we are thinking about symptoms without disease – PTSD and stuttering, and these are just two examples. To say that a person has medically unexplained symptoms is simply to acknowledge the lack of a clear-cut physical pathology – preferably macroscopic pathology – to explain them.[7] Over time, some of these symptoms will come to be decisively linked to defined pathological processes. Freud expressed the naturalistic belief that *all our provisional ideas will someday be based on an organic substructure … We take this possibility into account when we substitute special forces in the mind for special chemical substances.*[8] Other symptoms will probably continue to defy this kind of categorisation.

Linking symptoms to pathology is the bedrock of the medical model of diagnosis and treatment, but another way of justifying a treatment in the absence of a firm rationale is by empirical expediency – 'We don't know why this works, but trust me, it does work.' It is this latter approach that convinced Yealland, Rivers and Logue that they were all on the right path, even though the maps they were drawing were quite distinct. The scientific method tries to test claims to cure by requiring that the results of any particular treatment should be replicable in other contexts. This requirement elicits protests from alternative medicine practitioners, who argue that there is something that is 'unreplicable' in their treatments. It's easy to see why they might make such a claim, when we consider Yealland's bullying, Rivers's respectful listening and Logue's unusual physical contortions. Each man believed in his method but each merely foreshadowed the later finding that the factors that work in therapy for medically unexplained symptoms are related to qualities in the therapist and the patient, rather than characteristics of the therapy.[9]

Novel treatments open up the potential for 'hype' in response to the well-worn injunction to 'use it (any new treatment) while it still works'. In other words, the placebo effect is likely to be strong when a novel treatment is heavily endorsed by a treating doctor, and to weaken as evidence emerges that the treatment may not be very effective, if at all. If a doctor acts as a confident guide in unfamiliar territory, then it may seem foolish to ignore him or her if other doctors do not seem able to suggest a way out. In *The King's Speech*, Lionel Logue is portrayed as persuading King George to shake himself, roll around on the floor, sing and swear – all as part of his treatment. Anyone with a mind to criticise the treatment or to accuse Logue of abuse of the therapist–patient relationship could have made a strong case that Logue was a charlatan and not to be trusted. And yet the movie portrays a sincere and empathic therapist who succeeds about as well as anyone could expect – and certainly more than most other therapists at the time.

This forces us to ask whether it really matters exactly *how* a treatment works, provided that it actually does bring relief. The situation is a little like that of the small boy who, on being asked for directions, was unable to say where he was. When his questioner became annoyed because he could not put a name to their location, the boy's retort was, 'I may not know where I am, but I ain't lost.' Those words could be the motto for those who argue that their methods are successful in helping people to find their way out of illness territory without having first 'located' the diagnosis.

Is the mechanism of action of a successful treatment less important than the results? From the perspective of the individual patient and the individual doctor, who cares how the treatment works? If Jake could find a cure for his unpredictable intestinal tract, we can be pretty sure that he would not hesitate to take it.

There are two problems with this approach. The first is that ignorance of the underlying mechanism of illnesses and treatments limits the potential for progress in understanding a disease or syndrome better. It also limits our ability to predict possible adverse effects of treatment. Perhaps even more important, ignorance can promote useless and even dangerous treatments that go around in self-justifying circles.

Wonder cures are popular precisely because they promise to address life's painful or at least uncomfortable realities – that our bodies are imperfect and that many symptoms are relatively harmless but not easily explained. Wonder cures are so wonderful that even the knowledge that there is no active ingredient (in any biomedical sense) only partly reduces treatment effectiveness. We appear to have the capacity to recruit non-specific healing mechanisms of the kind that would normally facilitate recovery from a 'true' organic illness.

As John Saunders points out in Chapter 8, alternative medicine has rewritten the illness map for many people, with new or modified locations marked 'stress', 'immune system overload', 'Ayurvedic healing' and 'holistic therapy'. However, orthodox medicine is not free of blame when it comes to creating labels with dubious heuristic value. Patients are often given medical-sounding labels like 'fibromyalgia' or 'repetitive strain injury'. Just last week I saw a patient who now believes that she has fibromyalgia. She first became aware of her symptoms when her parents' marriage breakdown reached a point of bitter irreconcilability. Only her pain, the result of a recent sports injury, was able to distract them from their mutually assured destruction. Fifteen years later she sees four different types of physical therapists to treat the consequences of that injury. Another patient with minor injuries from what had been a terrifying, 'near miss' aeroplane accident was able to relinquish her pain symptoms only after the insurance company acknowledged the liability that they had previously denied.

This can be frustrating for the clinician who prefers to unroll a map with a clearly recognisable biomedical notation. We like to say, 'The signs were classical,' 'It was a typical presentation of glaucoma,' and 'Just as I suspected, that patient had an enlarged supraclavicular node.' An accumulation of clinical experience marks the map more and more clearly and the tools of evidence-based medicine provide a new perspective – a view of the whole terrain. If treatment needs a map, then evidence-based medicine is the view from the helicopter. (While the view from above can be useful, it has led to squabbles between pilots and foot soldiers. In particular, the foot soldiers like to point out that the terrain is tough, and the view on the ground takes in many important details that cannot be seen from a distance. Not only that, but when a request for information about the terrain is relayed to the helicopter, the message often comes back that the particular terrain in question has never been properly surveyed.)

When I compare the two maps – one prepared on the basis of evidence-based machine and one on the basis of my knowledge of an individual, what should I do about the inevitable mismatches? What risks am I (and my patient) willing to run by not chasing the diagnosis to a conclusion? Is a one-in-a-thousand chance of serious illness too great a risk? One in five hundred? One in fifty? What if other explanations for the illness experience seem to fit the patient more closely?

FINDING A WAY FORWARD

My last patient today is a junior doctor with an eating disorder. She can only manage a small amount of food each day. A busy and stressful job has left her unable to face another year of similar work. Her self-denial with food has become a symbol of her desire to save the world. Yesterday a high-achieving student described his disabling fatigue and a woman described to me some abdominal discomfort that she fears as evidence of serious gastrointestinal pathology. Another patient told me how regretful he is that his back pain has forced him onto a disability pension, even though there is only equivocal evidence of organic pathology. Each patient has developed ideas about a physical disorder that could explain their symptoms. Their explanatory map, however, does not match with mine.

As a doctor I assume that most of us, most of the time, wish not to be ill. Illness limits our normal activities and keeps us apart from family and friends. Illness can be expensive and time consuming. Perhaps the easiest thing for the doctor to do is to focus on the patient's physical complaints, take an orthodox medical history, conduct a physical examination, order tests and communicate the results. If there are no abnormalities, I can reassure the patient. If the symptoms persist, perhaps I can find a name from whatever is in fashion at the moment.

But the reality is that, for patients who seem to have a medically unexplained illness, I could also find out more about the reason for the discrepancy between our two maps, invalidating neither one nor the other. Working in a wider cultural and social milieu, Arthur Kleinman suggests that the physical expression of psychological disorder is not an aberration but may be the norm.[10] One of the challenges of treatment, therefore, is matching the doctor's map with that of the patient. Kleinman suggests that certain lines of questioning will help doctors to understand patients' health problems more easily. He suggests asking, 'What do you think the problem may be?' and 'What do you think may be the cause?' Such questions seem to contradict ideas of the doctor as expert, with a focus on somatic symptoms. However, there is evidence to suggest that emotional support matters more to patients with medically unexplained symptoms than a physical explanation for the symptoms.[11]

Perhaps because of this mismatch, therapists and patients continue to create maps labelled with syndromes and treatments for which there is little if any objective evidence. Ross[12] suggests that disease labels behave like 'infectious agents that, like microbes, have virulence factors, affect hosts with particular vulnerabilities, are disseminated through a variety of vectors and are promoted or inhibited by various components of social ecology'. With our map metaphor, we could say that illness labels aspire to be recognised place names on the official map.

Because of the inherent difficulty in managing medically unexplained symptoms, it is easy to understand why some doctors turn to the easy labels, but it could be argued that patients have enough pain or impairment of function without being weighed down by spurious diagnoses, inappropriate pain prescriptions and other physical interventions. The judicious use of the best available evidence is not as glamorous as becoming a self-styled 'expert' in chronic fatigue syndrome (CFS), IBS or fibromyalgia; books and websites devoted to CFS, IBS or fibromyalgia demonstrate that there is a buoyant market for such products.

Regeneration includes some useful observations on treatment in the absence of a clear diagnosis. Rivers was motivated by a genuine regard for the young men for whom he was responsible, and he saw each of them as an individual and as worthy of attention in his own right. He used what would later become standard treatment – respect, attentive listening, honest feedback, appropriate challenging and, above everything else, the willingness to travel alongside his young patients and to translate from his map to theirs and back again. Although the level of trauma that they had experienced was far greater than anything our patients might face today, the principles of treatment have not changed and the evidence base to support them has increased steadily.

A lingering question remains – does the kindness and understanding that Rivers showed to his young soldiers really qualify as 'treatment' or should there always be a biomedical diagnosis as a justification for what doctors do? The status of medically unexplained symptoms continues to raise questions: Are some varieties of the illness experience inherently more worthy of attention than others? What are the rights and responsibilities of doctors for making moral judgements about the status of different kinds of human distress? What are the limits of our medical responsibility for the well-being of our patients? What constitutes health?

Doctors cannot avoid making moral judgements that can have profound implications for the lives of their patients, yet biomedicine provides no language with which to examine or judge human behaviour. Like Yealland, Rivers and Logue, we rely on values that remain largely unexamined, and often unrecognised.

If there are basic human needs without which we cannot hope to flourish, either singly or within communities, then it should be possible to identify and draw together the values that address those needs. Our needs operate at many levels, or, to express it a little differently, our needs can be represented by many maps. Reducing symptoms and signs to their molecular causes does not imply that these constitute an adequate explanation of experience. It is merely one kind of map. Molecular, physical, emotional and social mechanisms all have a bearing on well-being, and all interact with one another. All are likely to be relevant to treatment.

Archie Cochrane is best known for his pioneering role in evidence-based medicine, but he is also well known for his stories of his own wartime experiences, and this is perhaps the best known among them:

> The Germans dumped a young Soviet prisoner in my ward late one night. The ward was full, so I put him in my room as he was moribund and screaming and I did not want to wake the ward. I examined him. He had obvious gross bilateral cavitation and a severe pleural rub. I thought the latter was the cause of the pain and the screaming. I had no morphia, just aspirin, which had no effect.
>
> I felt desperate. I knew very little Russian then and there was no one in the ward who did. I finally instinctively sat down on the bed and took him in my arms, and the screaming stopped almost at once. He died peacefully in my arms a few hours later. It was not the pleurisy that caused the screaming but loneliness. It was a wonderful education about the care of the dying. I was ashamed of my misdiagnosis and kept the story secret.[13]

Rather than being a misdiagnosis, Cochrane's experience is really just an example of how easy it is to allow one treatment map to obscure the others. Reductionism in medicine is the mindset that always moves toward a single level of explanation – in most cases, from the social to the cellular. While this kind of reductionism is undesirable, it must be remembered that it can also run in the opposite direction – from the cellular to the social as well as from the social to the cellular. Reductionism is reductionism because it privileges one kind of map. To do this is to limit treatment options by failing to recognise the many levels at which treatment occurs. Insulin and blood sugar levels may be vitally important on the map for the treatment of diabetes but, as every treating physician knows, the greatest long-term challenges in the management of diabetes relate to a patient's lifestyle – to work, recreation, self-care and relationships.

Writing in *The New York Times*[14] Anatole Broyard says that it is the task of the doctor to 'usher the patient out of the ordinary world into whatever place awaits him. The physician is the patient's only familiar in a foreign country.' Continuing his metaphor of countries, terrains and maps, Broyard says: 'Not every patient can be saved, but his illness may be eased by the way the doctor responds to him.... He has little to lose and much to gain by letting the sick man into his heart. If he does, they can share, as few others can, the wonder, terror and exaltation of being on the edge of being, between the natural and the supernatural.'

The wise physician 'comprehends', or draws together, all of the maps, spreading them out in clear view on the treatment table and consulting them as appropriate for the task at hand. Whether they are labelled 'cure', 'care' or 'comfort', while even a single map rests on the table, the professional responsibility to guide, to orientate or simply to be with the patient remains.

REFERENCES

1 Broyard A. Doctor talk to me. *The New York Times (Health)*. New York, NY. 16 August, 1990. p. 6.
2 Barker P. *Regeneration*. New York, NY: Plume; 1993. p. 227.
3 Yealland LR. *Hysterical Disorders of Warfare*. London: MacMillan and Co Ltd; 1918. pp. 7–8.
4 Sassoon S. *Sherston's Progress*. London: Faber & Faber; 1936. p. 51.
5 Bronowski J. *The Common Sense Of Science*. Cambridge, MA: Harvard University Press; 1978. p. 120.
6 Hooper T. *The King's Speech*. United Kingdom: Momentum Theatrical; 2010.
7 Kirmayer LJ, Groleau D, Looper KJ et al. Explaining medically unexplained symptoms. *Canadian Journal of Psychiatry*. 2004; **49**: 663–72.
8 Freud S. On narcissism: an introduction. In: J Strachey, editor. (Trans. J Strachey). *The Standard Edition Of the Complete Psychological Work Of Sigmund Freud*. London: Hogarth Press; 1957. p. 78.
9 Hubble MA, Duncan BL, Miller SD, editors. *The Heart & Soul Of Change: what works in therapy*. Washington DC: American Psychological Association; 1999.
10 Kleinman AL, Eisenberg L, Good B. Culture, illness, and care: clinical lessons from anthropologic and cross-cultural research. *Focus*, 2006; 4: 140–9.
11 Salmon P, Ring A, Dowrick CF, *et al*. What do general practice patients want when they present medically unexplained symptoms, and why do their doctors feel pressurized? *Journal of Psychosomatic Research*. 2005; **59**: 255–60.
12 Ross S. 'Memes' as infectious agents in psychosomatic illness. *Annals of Internal Medicine*. 1999; **131**: 867–71, p. 867.
13 Cochrane A. *One Man's Medicine*. London: BMJ Books; 1989. p. 82.
14 Broyard A. Doctor talk to me. *The New York Times (Health)*. New York, NY. 16 August, 1990. p. 9.

CHAPTER 7

The paradox of placebo – real and sham in medicine

RAIMO PUUSTINEN AND PEKKA LOUHIALA

In his novel *The Egyptian* Mika Waltari depicts how an ancient physician Senmut was once visited by a female patient who 'sighed and moaned and lamented over her many afflictions'.[1] After listening to the patient the physician

> wrote a line in ancient characters copied from a worn papyrus roll, then poured oil and wine into a mixing bowl and soaked the paper in it until the ink had been dissolved by the wine. Then he poured the liquid into the earthenware jar and gave it to the spice dealer's wife as a medicine, telling her to take some of it whenever head or stomach began to pain her.

When the woman left the surgery, Senmut's son gave a baffled look at his father who seemed embarrassed, coughed once or twice and then said:

> Many diseases can be cured with ink that has been used for powerful invocation.' He said no more aloud, but muttered to himself after a time, 'At least it can do the patient no harm.'

In the case above the physician deliberately prescribed a treatment of which he himself seems to have doubted the efficacy. Administering non-effective treatment may also happen inadvertently, as the following real-life case vignette from contemporary medical practice demonstrates.

> One of the authors of this essay (RP) was once working in an emergency ward when a middle-aged man with a severe pain in his left flank was rushed in. It turned out that the patient's pain was due to a kidney stone. The physician told the nurse to get injectable indomethacin. The nurse returned with a syringe filled with opaque liquid. The physician confirmed that the liquid was the substance required and the nurse nodded her head. The physician then injected the liquid into the patient's vein and assured him that the pain will disappear within a minute or two. Soon the patient's expression relaxed, he grasped the physician's arm and thanked him with tears in his eyes. The pain was gone.
>
> The physician went to the office to write notes. There was an empty box of injectable indomethacin on the table. When the physician dropped the box into a bin he noticed a small bottle in the box containing white powder. He realised that the inexperienced young nurse had not mixed the indomethacin powder into the saline he had injected into the patient.

In this case the physician had acted in good faith when assuming that the substance he injected into the patient would help him. Although the substance given was biologically inert, the patient benefited from the treatment. How should we understand this phenomenon? Yet there are cases when the patient's problem may be relieved even without receiving any treatment, as the following real-life example exemplifies:

> A couple of years ago the other author of this essay (PL) had a common cold with exceptional tiredness and occasional irregular pulse. This led him to consult a doctor, who turned out to be his former student. After a careful clinical examination and studying the electrocardiogram (ECG) the doctor explained that the results were normal and there were only a few benign extrasystoles seen in the ECG. Suddenly, the tiredness went away and the patient felt well again.

In this case merely visiting a physician and being acknowledged, heard, understood, comforted and reassured proved to be beneficial. This, indeed, is a common experience among physicians and patients alike.

These examples suggest that there is more involved in medical treatment than administering definitive biological measures to affect a given disease process. In contemporary medical literature we describe a beneficial outcome of a treatment that cannot be fully explained by biomedical concepts as a placebo effect. The concepts of placebo and placebo effect, however, are somewhat problematic in their current medical use. The word 'placebo' is applied to biologically inert treatments, such as the ineffective preparations given to control groups in clinical trials. The problem we face here is if placebo is inert by definition, how can we then speak of a placebo effect? In what follows we shall discuss the roots of this self-contradictory use of these terms and examine ways to overcome this ongoing conceptual confusion in medical thinking and literature.

TREATMENT AND CARE

In medicine we like to think that we treat the disease and care for the patient. For example, we use expressions such as 'surgical treatment' or 'pharmacological treatment' and 'palliative care' or 'elderly care'. It seems, then, that when we are using the concept of treatment we mean therapeutic measures that are based on scientific studies and that are intended to adjust injured or diseased bodily structures and functions to normal, as when we give penicillin to cure pneumonia. When we use the concept of care we indicate measures that are targeted to soothe and alleviate whatever problems the patient has. For example, in our story of Rachel's diabetes she receives medical treatment to adjust her blood glucose to normal levels. When we cannot provide restoration to normal, as in our story of Geoff's paralysis, we try to provide care for the patient in order to alleviate the consequences of the disease and to help him to continue his life with as little discomfort as possible. Yet care is more or less present in all medical treatment and cannot be excluded from it even in the direst occasions such as emergency operations on severely injured patients. With the concept of care we refer here to the ability of doctors (and the whole clinical team) to calm, reassure and comfort their patients. In medical literature we tend to place this ability under the rubric 'the art of medicine' apart from 'science' in medicine. How do the concepts of placebo and placebo effect fit into this general picture?

Placebo and placebo effect

The word 'placebo' (from Latin *placeo*, 'to please') entered the medical vocabulary in the late 18th century. Motherby's *New Medical Dictionary* of 1791 gives it a definition as 'a commonplace method or medicine'. The meaning of the word, however, changed in only a couple of decades. In 1808 *The Philadelphia Medical Dictionary* defines placebo as 'an epithet given to any medicine adapted more to please than benefit the patient'. This change of meaning of the concept of placebo is attributed to the critical impetus of the Enlightenment on contemporary medical thinking.[2]

The phrase 'placebo effect' appeared in the medical literature in the early 20th century but it became widely used only after Henry Beecher's article 'The powerful placebo', published in 1955.[3] This work was the first meta-analysis of comparative studies where biologically inert medications were used to differentiate the effects of the medicinal compound under scrutiny.

Since the 1950s the use of randomised controlled trials in medical research has become commonplace to the point of being considered as the gold standard in contemporary clinical research. In research settings the control groups receiving placebos, that is, biologically inert substances, are called 'placebo groups'. The concept of a placebo effect is, in turn, used to denote observed changes in the placebo groups. The effect of the treatment is calculated by extracting the effect observed in the placebo group from that observed in the treatment group.

It seems to us, then, that the notion of placebo effect has today two main meanings: observed changes in the placebo group of a randomised double-blind trial and effects observed in an individual patient in a therapeutic setting where the beneficial outcome cannot be explained by our current biological understanding. In the medical literature these two meanings are often treated as equal while they are, in fact, two essentially different issues. That is, the aim of a clinical trial is to find an answer to a scientific question, while the aim in a clinical encounter is to help the patient. In a clinical trial the patient is told that after randomisation he or she may end up in a placebo group, and informed consent is obtained. It may be emphasised here that although it is well known that there are serious drawbacks in the consent process and patients' understanding of the principles of randomisation, this does not change the fact that expectations in a clinical trial are not the same as in an individual therapeutic setting. In the case of the latter both the physician and the patient expect and hope that the treatment will be effective, while in the former all the participants of the research agree that there may be no beneficial outcome for the patient whatsoever.

Redefining placebo

Now that placebo has, by definition, no effect, how can we then speak of a placebo effect? And if placebo does have some effect after all, how can this phenomenon be understood? Let us exemplify the difficulties in trying to answer these questions by considering Shapiro and Shapiro's definition of placebo in their book *The Powerful Placebo: from ancient priest to modern physician*[4] as

> any treatment ... that is used for its ameliorative effect on a symptom or disease but that actually is ineffective or is not specifically effective for the condition being treated.

The placebo effect is then defined as

> primarily the nonspecific psychological or psychophysiological therapeutic effect produced by a placebo, but may be the effect of spontaneous improvement attributed to the placebo.

If we replace the word 'placebo' with its definition above in the last sentence, we end up with the following:

> therapeutic effect produced by any treatment ... that actually is ineffective or is not specifically effective for the condition being treated ... but may be the effect of spontaneous improvement attributed to the [treatment].

The first part makes no sense and the second part limits the therapeutic result to spontaneous improvement only and rules out all other components of the therapeutic encounter.[5] It is also noteworthy that Shapiro and Shapiro, similar to many other authors, tried to get away with this confusion by using the term 'nonspecific' when addressing the alleged result of the placebo effect. This, however, refers only to the fact that we do not know what takes place in a therapeutic encounter when the patient feels better despite having not received any biologically plausible treatment.

Some authors have tried to explain the placebo effect by referring to the context of the clinical encounter. Miller and Kaptchuk,[6] for example, suggested that the placebo effect should be reconceptualised as 'contextual healing'. By this they refer to the context of the clinical encounter, as distinct from the specific treatment interventions containing factors such as the environment of the clinical setting, the communication between patient and clinician and the rituals of treatment.

Also Moerman[7] referred to the context when he suggested that much of what is called the 'placebo effect' is a special case of the 'meaning response', which is defined as the physiological or psychological effect of meaning in the origins or treatment of illness. When such effects are positive, they include most of the things that have been called the 'placebo effect' and, when they are negative, they include most of what has been called the 'nocebo effect'. Meaning response is attached to the prescription of active as well as inert medications and treatments.

These suggestions manage, in our opinion, to address the key issues but are, however, not readily usable for the replacement of the concepts of placebo and placebo effect. Contextual healing refers to the whole context of the therapeutic encounter that is, by necessity, always contextual in one way or another. Meaning response catches, in our opinion, the essence of the phenomenon but the content of these concepts have not, to our reading, been analysed in depth nor have they been adopted for wider use in medical writing.

Care effect

We have suggested elsewhere[8] that the concept of placebo should be limited to a research context only. The term 'placebo' would refer, then, only to the procedures and substances that are used as biologically inert controls to active treatments in medical research. When inert substances or treatments are used in clinical practice, they should not be called 'placebos'. If a treatment is ineffective for a particular patient or problem, let it be called an ineffective treatment.

There is no reason to adopt a particular concept for that in the clinical context even in the case where an inert treatment has been administered deliberately, and especially so when there is a broad consensus in contemporary medicine that such practice is unethical.[9]

To replace the phrase 'placebo effect' we have suggested the phrase 'care effect', which refers to the phenomena that take place within both research settings and clinical consultations leading to beneficial therapeutic outcomes in cases when the medical treatment given cannot explain those outcomes in full.

The reason we suggested this is that in addition to being obscure, the terms 'placebo' and 'placebo effect' have pejorative connotations regardless of what has been written about their importance, existence and supposed mechanisms. The language associated with placebo is, in general, negative. Placebos are described with terms such as 'dummy' or 'sham' and placebo effect as 'suggestion', 'noise' or 'bias'. Expressions such as, 'It is merely a placebo effect,' are common when denoting a positive outcome of a treatment that the speaker does not consider theoretically plausible.

Contrary to that, terms such as 'care' and 'caring' carry positive connotations (for example, concern and responsibility).[10] They are free of the burden that placebo has obtained as referring to something that is somehow unreal, whereas the patient's experience of having been cared for is always real. We believe that this experience is potentially evoked in all therapeutic encounters, providing that the patient is not unconscious or severely demented. It follows that when there are therapeutic outcomes that cannot be fully explained in terms of the supposed mechanisms of, for example, a pharmacological treatment, they may be considered as a consequence of being acknowledged, heard, understood, comforted and assured within a clinical encounter, that is, being cared for. That experience may be evoked in a clinical trial, too, but, as noted above, clinical context and research context are fundamentally different settings. In a clinical trial, the care effect may be considered as a confounding factor, not an ally, as in clinical medicine.

If the essence of the care effect is in the patient's experience of being cared for, let us ask how that experience is evoked in a clinical encounter.

Care as dialogue

The standard explanation of the mechanisms of the placebo effect offered in contemporary medical literature is that it is a psychological phenomenon. In this respect our claim that the care effect is an experiential phenomenon also falls into the realm of psychology to be explored. Yet to say that this phenomenon is a psychological one faces at least two theoretical problems. First, psychologists themselves seem to disagree on the nature of psyche or mind. We get different answers if we ask, say, a behaviourist, a cognitive psychologist, a neuropsychologist or a gestalt psychologist what is mind and how it should be examined. It appears, then, that when we physicians say that the placebo effect is a psychological phenomenon we do not say very much. Perhaps it is for us physicians just another way to try to get rid of the problem. Yet the problem does not disappear by just wrapping it up and placing it outside the door waiting for someone to come and put it out of sight.

Second, claiming that the placebo or care effect is a psychological phenomenon indicates that mind is somehow separated from the body (otherwise how would the one effect the other?). That leads us to the perennial and unresolved question of what constitutes mind and how it is related to the body. If we mean that mind is a non-material entity affecting the material body, we end in philosophical problems of such a scale that we do not wish to succumb to them within the realms of this essay (or elsewhere for that matter). But if explaining the placebo effect as a psychological phenomenon does not suffice, what then will? Let us try to outline one possible approach to the problem.

We may consider healing as a joint activity between a patient and a healer who share a common goal: to help the patient with his or her problems and ailments. Yet mere benevolent intention to help does not take the participants of a therapeutic encounter very far. What is also required for a successful therapeutic process is a shared understanding of the nature of the problem and the means needed to cure it. For example, if a patient with a prolonged low-back pain is told by the physician that his problem is a psychological one and he should start taking antidepressants and should see a psychotherapist, the patient may walk out of the clinic deeply offended if he is convinced that he does not have any psychological problems whatsoever and that his problem is purely a bodily one. On the other hand, if the physician shows the patient a magnetic resonance imaging (MRI) picture on his low back with indications of a compressed nerve root, the patient may readily accept that explanation and consent to the treatment plan offered, regardless of whether the physician's interpretation of the MRI picture has anything to do with the patient's pain in the first place. Now there is a shared understanding between the physician and the patient of the nature of the patient's problem and that creates trust for the patient towards the physician and hope that he will benefit from the treatment. This trust and hope may help the patient to feel better already on his way out of the clinic, or even during the encounter: 'I feel so much better now, doctor, that the reason for my pain has finally been found.' That trust and hope would most probably affect the patient's estimate of the severity of his pain for the better if he had been interviewed about it before and after the consultation. To call that change in perceived pain a placebo effect is, in our opinion, problematic because it indicates that the change is somehow unreal, an outcome of sham, dummy, suggestion, noise or bias in medical treatment. The fact that the patient feels better through understanding, trust and hope that is shared with the doctor is not sham or dummy; it is real.

Trust and hope are also present in cases when patients consent to medical examination and treatment even when they do not fully understand what is going on. Seeking medical advice, accepting the diagnosis and consenting to treatment indicate trust in doctors and hope for cure. Yet the problem of the care effect cannot be reduced merely to receiving and understanding medical facts, as we can see in our case stories about Liz and Jen who were both well informed about what was going on and still felt more or less confused and lost with their condition. What more, then, is at stake here?

In medical education we are instructed to 'listen to the patient', or to 'see the patient as a person'. These instructions, we believe, address the issue correctly but only partially. To be able to discern a patient's problem requires, obviously, listening to what the patient says at the surgery, reading between the lines and observing his or her physical expressions, as every seasoned clinician is able to tell. The problem in the clinical encounter from the physician's point of view is that what the patient says can be quite remote from what we have been taught to consider medically relevant. On the other hand, patients often refrain from telling clinically relevant facts, such us the amount of alcohol they actually consume. Furthermore, if the patient's often irrational fears and worries do not become audible during the consultation, the issues that the patient holds as important may never be dealt with in the clinical dialogue. The patient may leave the clinic after receiving appropriate medical information and proclaim that 'the doctor didn't listen to me' or 'he found nothing in the test results' or 'she was just staring at her computer'. The patient may then end up seeing, say, an acupuncturist, and we hear how he or she 'took me seriously' and 'found the reason for my pains in my blocked energy channels'. In cases such as this we may assume, however, that there has been more going on than just examining the patient's pulse to arrive at the diagnosis of a blocked energy channel and sticking needles in various parts of his or her body in complete silence. Whatever the patient experienced with the therapist we may assume that his or her plea was somehow acknowledged and shared, no matter how irrational that may have been from a medical viewpoint (or from the acupuncturist's viewpoint for that matter). Once the patient sensed shared understanding with the therapist he or she gained hope for recovery through the treatments he or she agreed to receive. That trust and hope together with the experience of being heard may help him or her feel better with his or her ailment, at least for a while. That outcome we would rather call a care effect than a placebo effect.

If the root of creating a care effect lies in a dialogical relationship between the patient and the healer, we may add here that the care effect does not necessarily require another person to be physically present. Let us think of a situation where a person feels ill and she takes some homeopathic pills that she has purchased from a homeopathic pharmacy. From a biological point of view, the preparation can have no effect on the patient whatsoever. But the patient nevertheless feels better after taking the medicament. Why is this so? It may be possible, of course, that it may be due to spontaneous improvement, as Shapiro and Shapiro have suggested. However, we cannot ignore the fact that in the patient's belief system homeopathic remedies may be beneficial (why would she otherwise bother to purchase and use them?). While the remedy itself contains a promise of cure, it needs to be administered in order to gain anything from it. In this setting the patient may say that she does not need to see a homeopath or a physician because 'I am treating myself'. To treat oneself is also a dialogical relationship where 'I' and 'myself' are the participants of that dialogue, negotiating the diagnosis and the treatment of choice to get better. This is precisely what Jake in our story did when declining medical help and taking peppermint oil to control his symptoms.

We have now positioned the care effect in the clinical dialogue within which the patient's problems have been acknowledged and shared with a physician in a living dialogue. That dialogue may evoke mutual understanding, trust and hope, elements that we consider as constituents of the experience of being cared for or the care effect. Let us see now how this phenomenon may be discerned in our patient stories.

Liz is visiting a gynaecologist for a colposcopy. The clinic has paid attention to soothe the patients' anxiety with carefully chosen furniture, nice colours and relaxing background music. Yet, Liz observes, 'None of the women waiting on these tasteful chairs looked comfortable.' The nurse calls Liz in and informs her that there will be students present as the clinic is part of a teaching hospital. Liz exercises her right to refuse and her refusal is accepted 'coldly'. When Liz meets the doctor she receives instructions and explanations in a 'brusque and perfunctory manner'. The doctor talks Liz through the procedure with warnings, explanations and advice on what is taking place during the examination. But 'she did not meet Liz's eye'. The event unfolds through performing technical procedures and delivering one-way information. In this story we are witnessing a technically well-conducted medical treatment where the patient's hopes are met through not letting the students attend and talking the patient through the procedure by delivering a set of medical facts. No dialogue, however, develops to make audible the fears and worries of the patient. The patient tolerates the discomforts of the event and tries to cope with them with some dry humour.

Jen has been diagnosed as having lung cancer. She is now receiving chemotherapy, which is making her sick. She has painful ulcers in her mouth. She is vomiting. She is having bouts of uncontrolled diarrhoea. One morning her hair is gone. She feels humiliated; her body has let her down. She feels that 'nobody has warned her it might happen'. Yet she has been told about her condition by the doctor with a 'kind face' and the nurse who made her a cup of tea and who measured her for a wig, reassuring her that her hair will grow back.

In both of these stories trust and hope are indicated by the fact that both Liz and Jen have consented to medical examination and treatment. But we feel that something is missing. To have a nicely decorated clinic and to provide accurate medical information does not seem to suffice. We assume that both of the patients feel that they have been well cared for. But would they have felt more so if their fears and worries had been brought into the dialogue alongside or even instead of them receiving a stream of plain medical facts?

In Geoff's story we sense an air of resignation. He stays in a single 'not too clinical' room with white walls. These adjustments may bring him a sense of comfort for the days that he has left to live. He is also receiving medical treatment with antidepressants, which are 'beginning to work', as the nurse observes. Also the physiotherapist is 'pleased with him'. No dialogue evolves, just a blink in the eye when Jen touches the patient. From the medical point of view it is time to consider sending Geoff back home.

In Jake's story we learn that he suffers from an inflammatory bowel disease with moderate to severe symptoms. Yet he plainly refuses any medical treatment. 'I don't want any more tubes stuck up and through me … I don't want any more of those bloody tests and … any bloody pills either.' Whatever had happed in the clinic previously has upset him to the point that he 'won't let them touch' him again. He insists that it is his body, he does not want to feel a 'freak' and he is not going back 'for more of that'. Whatever 'that' consists of, we have no way of knowing. All we can tell is that he would rather suffer his symptoms and try to cope with them by taking peppermint oil rather than go back to the clinic for further tests and treatments. Whatever has been discussed in the clinic, no mutual understanding on how his condition should be treated has developed between Jake and those attending him. Clinical dialogue has turned into repulsive experience, keeping Jake away from doctors.

Rachel has her diabetes treated to the point that she can live a rather normal life. The problem is with other people in her life who cannot cope with her illness: her mother and her teacher. Rachel's doctor does not get involved with those problems beyond writing a letter of reassurance that there is no medical reason whatsoever not to participate in the normal activities and joys of life. That letter was initiated by Dax, the nurse who 'can sort things out'. And not only that, but she has taken the responsibility of Rachel's well-being to the point that Rachel's mother can phone her 'any time you like'. Her willingness and ability to acknowledge Rachel's mother's fears and worries and to bring them into a dialogue with her may eventually calm the mother and help the family cope better with Rachel's diabetes. That may also be beneficial in terms of influencing her long-time blood glucose balance. Would we, really, call such an outcome a placebo effect?

CONCLUSION

The concept of placebo is not needed in clinical medicine. An ineffective treatment is ineffective whether or not it has been administered purposefully or unintentionally. Placebos – defined as biologically inert substances or procedures – are needed only as controls in randomised clinical trials.

When a patient reports that he or she feels better after receiving a treatment that should not theoretically produce such an outcome we suggest the concept of care effect to denote that phenomenon. The care effect is constituted by the patient's experience of being cared for. That experience is contained within the dialogical relationship between a patient and a healer where the patient feels that his or her plea has been answered and where both participants share the same understanding of the nature of the patient's problem and the means to cure or alleviate it.

By analysing a therapeutic event as a goal-directed dialogic activity we may gain deeper understanding of what takes place during a clinical encounter to trigger the experience of being cared for. Dialogical phenomena cannot, even in principle, be addressed with biological concepts and methods. They fall into the realm of social sciences and humanities to explore. Medical humanities is a methodological solution for medicine to explore in depth its core event, the therapeutic encounter, and the manifold phenomena present in its course.

REFERENCES

1 Waltari M. *The Egyptian*. Porvoo: Werner Söderström Osakeyhtiö; 1983. p. 10.

2 Schiller F. An eighteenth century view of the placebo effect. *Clio Medica*. 1984; **19**: 81–6.

3 Beecher H. The powerful placebo. *JAMA*. 1955; **159**: 1602–6.

4 Shapiro AK, Shapiro E. *The Powerful Placebo: from ancient priest to modern physician*. Baltimore, MD: The Johns Hopkins University Press; 1997. p. 1.

5 Moerman D. *Meaning, Medicine and the 'Placebo Effect'*. Cambridge: Cambridge University Press; 2002.

6 Miller F, Kaptchuk T. The power of context: reconceptualizing the placebo effect. *J R Soc Med*. 2008; **101**: 222–5.

7 Moerman D. op. cit. Also: Moerman DE, Jonas WB. Deconstructing the placebo effect and finding the meaning response. *Ann Intern Med*. 2002; **136**: 471–6.

8 Louhiala P, Puustinen R. Rethinking the placebo effect. *Medical Humanities*. 2008; **34**; 107–9.

9 AMA 2006: American Medical Association Council on Ethical and Judicial Affairs. Placebo use in clinical practice [cited 30 July 2013. Available at: www.ama-assn.org/ama1/pub/upload/mm/369/ceja_recs_2i06.pdf.

10 Tudor Hart J, Dieppe P. Caring effects. *Lancet*. 1996; **347**: 1606–8.

8

Considering the alternatives: or, who is the medicine man?

JOHN SAUNDERS

Nahkira Harris was nine years old when she died in February 1992.[12] She had wasted away before her parents' eyes, who, said the prosecutor at Nottingham Crown Court, buried their heads in the sand of their own intransigence, pride and fanaticism and their own perceived purity. Like Rachel in our story, Nahkira had diabetes. But Nahkira didn't receive insulin. Her parents were believers in homeopathy. They removed their daughter from hospital after diagnosis, angry at the doctors' insistence that the only effective treatment was insulin. Their general practitioner could have saved the girl's life, contended the defence counsel; but he had attended instruction at the Society of Homeopaths. Six weeks after diagnosis, Nahkira was dead. For her there was no Dax, no parent who would promote her interests, no doctor on her side: only a verdict of manslaughter. The ancient 'wisdom' of signatures had killed her.

THE OLD ART

Medicine men constitute the oldest professional class in the evolution of society.[3] With stripes on his limbs, a large pair of antlers on his head and covered in an animal skin, the oldest known portrayal of a medicine man can be seen in the Trois Frères cave in the Pyrenees. It dates to about 15,000 BC. Numerous prehistoric skulls provide evidence of the operation of trephining (cutting a hole in the skull). The treatment was widespread and survived into the 20th century, where it has been recorded as therapy for epilepsy, headache and insanity or simply in order to promote longevity. The practice of medicine is as long as humankind itself. People have always tried to overcome or control distress, disease and death. Yet medicine is also described as the youngest science. What we know as medicine today embraces *scientific* medicine: the application of general laws to human beings in the same way that engineers apply general laws to the construction of bridges.[4] The distinguished American physician Lewis Thomas entitled his biographical reflections *The Youngest Science*.[5] Thomas relates an anecdote when he was totally involved in the 'science of medicine'. A guest speaker at a county medical society, the society president was telephoned during the society's annual meeting and he left to not return to the gathering. When he did return, Thomas asked what had caused him to leave. The president explained that an old woman had died and that he knew that her family was in distress and needed him. He said that he was sorry to have missed the evening but that some things cannot be helped. Thomas concludes, 'This was in the early 1950s, when medicine was turning into a science, but the old art was still in place.'

'The old art': for Thomas this was the concern for the suffering of a fellow human being, translated into practical action. The science, he seems to assert, is new – shockingly new to those of us accustomed to date medicine's transition to modernity somewhere in the nineteenth century, with the triumph of the new orthodoxy in Great Britain enshrined in the Medical Act of 1858. The story suggests that only in the last century or so has medicine really offered anything to reduce the mortality or morbidity of most sufferers. A few significant earlier discoveries stand out – antisepsis or anaesthesia or quinine – but mostly the story is one of ineffective interventions, sometimes with disastrous consequences.

TRADITIONAL AND SPIRITUAL

One of those features that contrasts modern orthodox medical practice with the practices of complementary and alternative medicine (CAM) is that the former is so eager to discard what it sees as outdated, while the latter is equally eager in its wish to emphasise its traditional roots. 'You could have the best of both worlds – better health naturally – by using the experience and wisdom from ancient cultures and combining modern science.' So ran the leaflet I was given, advertising a herbal remedy. Some complementary therapies place great emphasis on natural means, on their antique roots and on cultural origins – often linked to Eastern mysticism. The emphasis on traditional and ancient roots is an image-building aspect of unconventional therapies: Ancient China for herbal medicine and acupuncture, Ancient Egypt for aromatherapy, Ancient India and Native Americans for reflexology and so on. The emphasis on continuity is reassuring for many, but it carries no connection with efficacy. It is not difficult to think of traditional practices that are thoroughly harmful, however 'natural' be the products employed (for example, bloodletting and trephining). Moreover, orthodox surgeons do not reassure their patients by informing them that amputation has been practised for 2000 years before they remove an ischaemic limb. Is this linking of CAM practices to supposed ancient wisdom another aspect of the search for meaning in our daily lives? Is it part of an attempt to find comfort from ultimate meaninglessness by linking ourselves in a tradition that has continued for so long and, by implication will continue, an integration into a spiritualised humanity, of which we are both part and also that continues beyond us? 'Above all else, herbalism is the medicine of belonging, the direct experience of the whole healing of the part...To heal ourselves we must know ourselves, and ecology, spirituality, intuition and common sense tell us that we are all one. If our world is poisoned, so are we.'[6]

Complementary and alternative medicine is hard to define. The variety of practices is so wide, the extremes are so absurd, the claims and counter-claims are so contradictory, that finding a common thread presents challenges. Pietroni writes:

> The term 'alternative' or 'complementary' medicine is used as a catch all definition for anything not taught at a Western medical school. It is thus a definition by exclusion and as helpful a term as 'foreign.' An Englishman setting out to comment on 'foreigners' would be as accurate in his description of foreigners as most doctors are in their understanding of alternative therapies, and the Englishman's commentaries on foreigners would tell us more about the prejudices of being English than the characteristics of non-English people.[7]

HISTORICAL BACKGROUND

Old medicine or young medicine? Understanding the roots may aid our understanding of the status of current practice. In his magisterial historical study, Keith Thomas[8] points out that a large proportion of the population of Tudor and Stuart England depended on a mixture of common-sense remedies, based on an accumulated experience of nursing and midwifery, combined with inherited lore about the healing properties of plants and minerals. It also included certain types of ritual healing – with prayers, charms or spells. Some of these practices were doctrinally based. According to the doctrine of signatures, for example, every herb was stamped with a sign of its uses: Yellow blossom indicated a cure for jaundice or a root shaped like a foot indicated a remedy for gout. The theory gradually was forgotten and by the mid-18th century, the properties of herbs were regarded as inherent naturally. The concept of what has since been called psychosomatic disease was wider in the seventeenth century than now, for contemporary intellectuals exaggerated the power of the imagination.[9] The potentialities open to purely physical remedies were limited:

small wonder that psychosomatic healing flourished. The 17th century saw the beginning of the decline in some of the more outlandish theories. The triumph of the mechanical philosophy meant the decline of the animistic conception of the universe[10] that constitutes the basic rationale for magical therapy.

Of course, most people had never heard of Newton or Harvey. Folk medicine continued to flourish as a mixture of magic, common sense and a crude empiricism. Cowpox protecting against smallpox or digitalis are two of its successes. Numerous manuals described these remedies, written by both physicians and others. In some, remedies were organised into systems of self-care. Samuel Thomson (1769–1843), for example, built up a system of botanicals[11] that his disciples were to develop into physio-medicalism.[12] In science, physio-medicalism abandoned chemical or materialistic theories of life and substituted a physiology based on vitalism and on the inherent power of the body's vital force. Thomsonianism,[13] introduced into England by Isaiah Coffin, was anti-establishment and truly alternative. It never managed to persuade a body of orthodox practitioners to accept its practices or to modify its doctrine to enable any accommodation: hence its disappearance more than 80 years ago. Another systematiser was John Brown (1735–88) who published his doctrines in *Elementa Medicinae* (1780). Brown posited that disease was due to excess (sthenic) or, more often, defect of stimulation (asthenic). The treatment consisted of heroic doses of stimulating drugs, often with obvious fatal results. Brunonian methods were said to have killed more people than the French Revolution and Napoleonic wars taken together[14] (and attracted the attention of such luminaries as Goethe[15]). A more successful systematiser was another near contemporary of Brown and Thomson, Samuel Hahnemann (1755–1843).[16] Hahnemann embraced the vitalism of the one while moving to the opposite extreme in dosage of the other. In his *Organon der Heilkunde* (1810), Hahnemann revived the doctrine of signatures in a new guise: *similia similibus* or 'like cures like'. In this way, he links modern CAM practice back to mediaeval roots. He soon propounded a second law concerning the value of extremely small or infinitesimal doses. His third postulate was the doctrine of 'psora': All 'natural' chronic disorders except venereal diseases were manifestations of the psora – or itch. Homeopathy survived because of the intellectual accommodations that homeopathic physicians were able to make to Hahnemann's doctrines – and because of the failure of conventional physicians to demonstrate superior outcomes in the first half of the 19th century. Orthodox medicine of the time – founded on Galenic or other theories hardly less plausible or modern than those of alternatives – killed so many patients with their bleeding and purging that homeopathy was often a safer option. Osteopathy, now recognised by statute in the United Kingdom with its own regulatory body, has a similar origin. Andrew Still (1828–87)[17] initially set up as a magnetic healer, following the doctrines of Franz Mesmer. He later combined the theoretical elements of magnetic healing and bone setting into one doctrine: practically all diseases were due to displacements and to heal one needed to readjust the displaced segment into its proper place and let nature do its work. From the beginning, osteopaths used great freedom in selecting therapies. The history of both homeopathy and osteopathy is one of struggles between those promoting the original founder's doctrine and those concerned with a more empirical approach. Today, the clinical practice of osteopathy is largely grounded in the orthodox medical sciences and regulation removes it from the fringe to a position that is possibly both established and unorthodox.[18] It is too easy to caricature many alternative systems by quoting the founding figure: hardly more valid than judging mainstream medicine by quoting its mistaken prophets. Nevertheless, it is useful to note the twin roots of much alternative medicine in folk traditions (herbalism, and so forth) and/or a dominating founding figure (homeopathy, and so on). A well-regulated and yet unconventional practice such as modern osteopathy should not be classed with the quack, so graphically described by Young.[19] We may need to ask: Is (for example) osteopathy the doctrine that Andrew Still described? Or is it what osteopathy schools now teach? Or is it what osteopaths do? Or is it what osteopaths believe?

CAM's emphasis on positive health leads to a variety of practices that prevent disease but also merge with faddism and commercially promoted health preservers: macrobiotic diets to cure cancer, marathon running to avoid heart disease, vitamin capsules and aerobic dancing to control stress. Folk medicine has contributed to CAM systems such as homeopathy and the doctrine of signatures. It also persisted into the 20th century in simplified traditional form, especially in rural areas: There was an array of treatments for warts and a wort for every ill – St John's wort tea for bed wetting as well as coughwort, chillwort, liverwort, spleenwort and, for cleaning the womb after the menopause, motherwort.[20].

Keith Thomas's study emphasises the long link between religion and the treatment of disease. The break up of the mediaeval church aided an increasing variety in medical practice. Thus, Stahl's animism takes its roots from Halle pietism.[21] The doctrines of Thomson and Hahnemann owed much of their success to links with dissent of all kind: anti-unionism, anti-establishment, free trade and non-conformity. Even in the mid-19th century, orthodoxy offered little and homeopathy, for example, was equally or more successful with its freedom from adverse effects. In much the same way, faith healing, which may offer at least a powerful placebo to large numbers, may be more successful in a primitive society than modern medicine, which may benefit only a select few.[22] By the late 19th century, medical education in Britain was university linked and the universities espoused naturalism in science. The decline of dissent assisted the establishment of orthodox medicine. Pluralism in medical practice was produced by patronage and the need to please the patient.[23] The state backing for orthodoxy through the Medical Act of 1858 and its increasing success marginalised many alternative medical activities. It is no coincidence that a more sceptical age that questions political authority, debates the success of scientific medicine and champions a consumerist faith is also an age in which complementary therapies thrive.

CAM IN THE MODERN WORLD: A UK PERSPECTIVE

The extent of that thriving has been well documented and each year new surveys demonstrate the involvement of doctors in CAM (perhaps 30% of general practitioners in the United Kingdom) and of patients (probably a majority in those with many long-term, psychosomatic or incurable complaints). CAM sells itself by offering benefits beyond those of Thomas's 'old art' and for the sickest or most seriously ill it offers a hope that is not tempered by the harsh realities of evidence.

The sharp growth in CAM was the subject of comment more than 25 years ago[24] and has produced a succession of reports in both the United Kingdom and the United States. 'Even the no-nonsense Margaret Thatcher was a devotee of mystical electrical baths and Ayurveda therapy,' wrote Francis Wheen.[25]

> But she was a mere dabbler compared with more recent inhabitants of Downing Street. Cherie Blair found her devout Catholicism no impediment to flirtations with New Age spirituality, inviting a feng-shui expert to rearrange the furniture at No 10 and wearing a 'magic pendant' ... which has a 'matrix of specially cut quartz crystals' that surround the wearer 'with a cocoon of energy' to ward off evil forces .... [She] was introduced to an 86-year-old 'dowsing healer', Jack Temple, who treated her swollen ankles by swinging a crystal pendulum over the affected area and feeding her strawberry leaves grown within the 'electromagnetic field' of a Neolithic circle he had built in his back garden.

Does this matter? One commentator wrote:

> Down here in Bournemouth medicine has more fringes than a Victorian tablecloth .... Mind you, when an old dear with a tumour almost certainly guaranteed to respond to a smidgeon of melphalan takes herself off to North Carolina to live on selenium yeast, coffee enema, and pancreatin tablets in a brave attempt to neutralise human chorionic gonadotrophin production, one is entitled to feel that the contesseration of quacks, acupressurists, aurasoma therapists, Bach flower arrangers, dowsers, ecowitches, homeopathists, Kirlian photographers, naturopaths and radio ionic diagnosticians, whose talisman is to call proper doctors allopaths, has overstepped the mark. I suppose that in Thatcherite Britain there should be no complaint. If you have a good product it will sell.[26]

Sampson has described how human immunodeficiency virus (HIV) has produced huge opportunities for opportunist peddlers of pseudo-science.[27] As he says, the cast of players includes 'well meaning self-help groups, self-deluded and self-important dreamers with gossamer philosophies and outright charlatans'. A notorious example of the latter genre was finally discredited only in September 2008, when Matthias Rath, a promoter of 'micronutrient' pills, while denouncing conventional medicine for AIDS as being toxic and dangerous, was forced into dropping a libel action against the UK's *The Guardian* newspaper.[28] Rath's foundation had promoted its micronutrient products for AIDS, cancer, heart disease and stroke in South Africa, Spain, France, Russia, United Kingdom and the United States. Rath was criticised as an example of the worst excesses of the alternative therapy industry in an area of practice where evidence really does matter and where orthodox treatment really does make a difference.

Supporters of CAM will almost certainly argue that the above examples are no more typical of daily CAM practice than are the negligent practices, inappropriate treatments, unnecessary investigations and adverse drug effects in orthodox medicine. Moreover, it is inevitable that CAM is so broad that critical anecdotes will never be in short supply. Confusing accredited CAM practitioners with cranks, fraudsters and pedants with an aversion to truth is a cheap attack on a false target.

For Prince Charles, CAM has a vital role to play in 21st-century healthcare. His Foundation for Integrated Medicine aimed to capitalise on the experience with CAM around the world, using traditional, 'natural' approaches, which are 'coordinated' with orthodoxy.[29] For the prince, CAM is primarily complementary, not alternative, and it must be 'integrated' into our current ways of working. The Foundation, incidentally, has now been dissolved following a major scandal, although a 'College of Medicine' has arisen, phoenix like, out of its ashes, supported by several prominent figures in the British medical establishment.

Most CAM therapists claim to treat the 'whole person' even though the modality of treatment may affect only one part of the body – as in iridology, reflexology or chiropractic. This is often accompanied by references to Cartesian dualism.[30,31] References to Descartes' writings or analysis of what he wrote are never given. The impression is that Descartes postulated an unbridgeable gap between body and mind. He did not.[32]

CAM AND HOLISM

CAM claims to be holistic. Holism is a term first coined in 1926 by JC Smuts[33] and gave rise to dispute in the philosophy of biology. Smuts explicitly opposed vitalism, which was understood to be an immaterial 'vital force' or 'vital principle' possessed by living beings: 'A living organism is not an organism plus life, as if life were something different and additional to it.'

Nevertheless, even Smuts did not clearly define holism and by the fifth chapter of his book there are already nine defining statements.[34] Imprecision and distortion in its use have occurred since. Smuts was also opposing a view of mechanism in biology. Whereas holists frequently oppose mechanism by recourse to vitalism, Smuts stressed that the whole was more than the sum of its parts, but not (contra vitalism), something added to its parts. Smuts' project was to explain how evolution can be creative, that is, how higher levels of wholes (for example, life) emerge from lower levels (for example, matter).[35] Darwinian natural selection tells us only why the unfit failed to survive and not why living beings, either fit or unfit, ever came into existence.[36] Smuts and JS Haldane argued that parts changed when synthesised into a whole to function differently. In medicine, extreme holists would seem to suggest that no analysis of the whole person in terms of his or her parts will yield knowledge about the whole. This implies that description of the behaviour of the whole is possible, but a complete analysis of this behaviour is not possible and therefore should not be attempted. The success of mechanistic science is reason enough to reject this view, even if mechanistic explanations cannot fully specify wholes. Learning to assemble an engine does not tell us what a car is for, but it does tell us something about it.

An early critic of holism pointed out that holists and mechanists were opposed about different things:

> The mechanist is concerned with how to proceed to a construction which will represent as much about the universe as human beings with their limited range of receptor organs agree to accept. The holist has an incorrigible urge to get behind the limitations of our receptor organs and tell us what the universe is really like.[37]

A more moderate holist view may not suggest the need to eliminate mechanistic analysis, but may suggest that organised wholes occur at various levels, so mechanistic explanations must be given at that level. This demonstrates that mechanism and reductionism are different concepts, although almost always confused in holistic medicine.

We may modify the moderate holist view further to acknowledge the value of reductionism without accepting that such explanations can ever be complete. Things may exist in hierarchies or on different levels, but the laws governing a lower level may still possess valuable explanatory power. As Bunge puts it,[38] we may combine ontological pluralism (that is, the recognition of variety) with epistemological reductionism (that is, that higher levels can be partly explained in terms of lower ones). The holist protest against radical reductionism is surely necessary, although it is hardly a distinctive feature of the alternative medicine lobby. The claim of radical reductionism, that all of the concepts, hypotheses and theories concerning things at a given level can in principle be reduced to those referring to things belonging to some other level, may have been productive, especially in physics from 1600 to 1800, but even here it is no longer credible. Quantum electrodynamics, quantum mechanics and the relativistic theory of gravitation are not reducible to one another, if only because they deal with things of radically different kinds. Still less is this possible in biology, where phenomena emerge with properties at one level of organisation that are not present at other levels of organisation. Biological systems have no vital force or principle but they do have properties that are not predicted or predictable from chemical laws or theory. Life is not a chemical property, but the statistical regularities of biological systems involve chemicals doing things not predicted by chemical laws. Biochemistry sets the boundary conditions: biological laws are additional. Perception, imagination, emotion, memory and so on are not predicted by the simple function of nervous cells. Psychological function may be independent of neurological correlates and the laws of memory and perception can be worked out without recourse to neural laws. The capacity for abstraction and symbolism takes man beyond the world of immediate experience in a quest for meaning. Only man has authenticity. This is meta-biological emergence. Emergence is not an obscure notion and does not have to be either accepted on faith (holism) or rejected with contempt (radical reductionism).

Generally speaking holists pay little attention to the large literature on reductionism in biology, so the concept is used loosely. Hull,[39] for example, discriminates between ontological, methodological and theory reduction. The first asserts that organisms are 'nothing but' atoms, to which anti-reductionists contrast structured (that is, ordered) wholes. Methodological reduction concerns optimal strategies in science; theory reduction seeks to explain one theory in terms of another. For example, classical Mendelian genetics may be explained in terms of molecular biology. Such explanations are fruitful in the research programmes that surround scientific theories. Thus Tay-Sachs disease at the level of the whole patient is shown to be due to an enzyme deficiency at the biochemical level; this in turn may be shown to be due to an abnormal gene at the genetic or molecular biological level. Hence rationally based genetic counselling emerges.[40] Reductive explanations in medicine are marked by appeals to genetic, biochemical and physicochemical causes of disease features. They need not be strictly deductive, that is, their content distinguishes them, not their logical form. For example, we may say that smoking causes lung cancer. There is a large body of evidence to support this, but the epidemiological evidence does not permit a strictly deductive conclusion about the behaviour of the bronchial mucosal cell from the behaviour of populations. The content of this argument gives it explanatory power.

Holists insist on the multi-factorial nature of disease, but reductionism does not deny this. Max von Pettenkofer drank a vial of living cholera bacilli and did not suffer.[41] He therefore demonstrated that other factors besides bacterial ingestion were important – presumably, in this foolhardy experiment, the strength of the inoculum. There is neither evidence nor reason to believe that reductionistic medicine will fail to seek and find an actual multi-factorial mechanism. What holists are usually about, however, is an emphasis on psychosomatic mechanisms and the distinctiveness of every patient. But psychological states do not have to be strictly identical for generalisations to be made any more than all apples have to be the same size in order to generalise about apples. The more extreme claim that all disease is psychosomatic is even less defensible, for there is no sense in which rubella or motor neurone disease or a host of others are caused psychosomatically. Orthodox medicine has never denied causal relationships between mind and body: anger causes the face to flush and fever causes delirium. There is no reason why a psychological event could not cause a physical event if every psychological event is associated with a physical event. The mind/brain interaction may be poorly understood, but that is no reason to postulate spiritual forces – or to retreat to a dualistic view of mind and body that holism simultaneously claims to avoid.[42] Once again holism dresses up a simple but important truism – consider psychological factors in the cause and response to disease – as a distinctive contribution to medicine.

OBFUSCATION IN LANGUAGE

Richard Asher wrote:[43]

> 'Any reasonable doctor … takes into account what the patient's home is like, what sort of family he has, and whether he is rich or poor. If Mr Jones lives in one room with five children, two cats and a drunken slatternly wife, any sensible doctor would not order him to rest at home with two-hourly feeds of steamed custard. Nobody would be the slightest bit impressed if anyone explained the obvious thing in a plain way, but if you follow my instructions and 'consider the patient as a psycho-dynamic whole, viewed as a socio-economic unit integrated within the cultural framework of his environmental and psychobiological relationships', then everybody will be deeply impressed.… The use of these key words lends an impressive and nebulous air of human profundity to your utterances and conveys that ordinary doctors are unsympathetic and remote beings with no interest in their patients' feelings.'

On the other hand, this seems to avoid defining what treatment is aiming to achieve. If Mr Jones is suffering from the debilitation of a recent infective illness, two-hourly custard feeds and some rest may suffice to return him to his daily activity as the family breadwinner. But Mr Jones's problems may go further and his hopes for therapy may be more ambitious. His debilitation may have its roots in a combination of bacterial, nutritional, psychological and social factors. Restoring Mr Jones to health will take more than custard and rest, or even antibiotics, custard and rest.

The language of 'holism' may do CAM a disservice. A willingness to consider the wider context of a patient's well-being may not be, and indeed is not, an exclusive preserve of the CAM practitioner and many CAM therapies, such as homeopathy, herbs or acupuncture may be offered in the same way as a course of penicillin.

Nevertheless, the rhetoric of CAM is generally far more sympathetic to a broader notion of health and to a wider use of words such as 'healing' or 'wholeness'. These considerations are, I would hazard a guess, one reason why CAM so often seems to touch on that area labelled 'the human condition' with its associated questions of, 'What is man?' or, 'What does it mean to be really human?' Such abstractions have no clear answers. That does not make them meaningless. The quest for meaning and the hallowing of human life are human pursuits of the most profound kind, engaging thinkers, writers and artists of every variety. Both physical and psychological health promote the purpose of life: they are not ends in themselves. Health is to be spent, just as money is. CAM is more sympathetic to such a view and to that degree has lessons for orthodox practice.

Modern scientific medicine is based on evidence that is graded according to its quality. The best quality evidence is usually stated to be the meta-analysis of double-blind randomised controlled trials. Recruitment to such trials can vary from a highly homogeneous group of participants to the pragmatic approach of recruiting everyone with the condition under study. In both cases there are problems of applying the trial's conclusions. In the first case, extrapolating data from a group of individuals of similar age, freedom from co-morbidities (and so on) to the patient who is older, sicker (and so forth) may not be justified. In the second case, the pragmatic study may show that the whole group benefit on balance, but there may be subgroups within the all-inclusive population who benefit more, or less or not at all. Subgroup analysis often cannot detect this. The trial is essentially an exercise in experimental epidemiology and its application to the individual patient may be inappropriate. CAM, by contrast, emphasises the individual in its treatment selection, promotes extensive personal attention and uses healing rituals. Treatment protocols, randomisation, double-blind conditions and use of placebo controls distort the 'holistic' therapeutic milieu of CAM, according to many of its practitioners. This may lead to inaccurate conclusions. Mozart or Mahler, Scarlatti or Sibelius, will not have the same effect on all individuals. A randomised trial would not be an appropriate technique to determine their value in promoting positive health. Rather any such conclusion would be based on individual reports. Perhaps this would be a better model for CAM: a variety of techniques with healing potential for individuals whose utility is closer to that of the novel or sonata than to the chemistry laboratory. Survival and spread of a particular technique may expand in the same way as the popularity of a piece of literature or music. Not all patients will like the odour of the particular aromatherapy, but the benefit to some individuals from the technique may be real. Personalised individual approaches may lead to healing, where healing means more than cure of a physical pathology. It is not whether CAM 'works' but what it means to say that it works. From the perspective of medical humanities that will be more than the double-blind randomised trial or even the qualitative study can demonstrate.

ADJUNCTIVE TREATMENTS

This brings us back to definitions and to the diversity of the interventions that fall under the CAM umbrella, as well as those that could but generally do not. In many children's wards in hospital, play therapists are routinely employed; clinical trials have been mounted on bibliotherapy; elsewhere music therapists and dance therapists make their contribution. Happy music[44] on prescription? Humour[45] therapy? At first, the idea of playing or reading or music making or music listening or joking or dancing as medical treatments appears odd. Ordinary experience, however, tells us that these activities do enrich our lives – why else would we promote them? To that degree, they make us healthier, better integrated and fuller people. If sick, they may support us in our recovery, encouraging us to make interventions such as becoming more active after a surgical procedure or encouraging us to partake in activities that assist our recovery from a psychiatric illness. They do not replace our ordinary treatments. Yet patients recover faster after surgery if nursed in wards with windows that let in daylight. Gardens are good for recovery. So perhaps we could speak of daylight therapy or horticultural therapy. On a bigger scale, many of us do believe that civic design and good architecture lead to better communities and yet we do not demand controlled trials in order to prove this. Such interventions in the way we live when either sick or well are often beyond the measuring rod of the conventional trial. The range of the intervention that may help may be too individualised to assess: Which music? Which sort of book? Which plants? What sort of humour? Windows that look out on what? The parallel with more conventionally understood CAM is obvious. Even in CAM, do we believe that we are taking complementary 'medicine' (aromatherapy) every time that we buy a product containing aloe vera?

Perhaps the most obvious, yet in some ways most extraordinary, example of a health-promoting intervention is laughter. Greenfield[46] points out that while laughter is a marvellous way of coping with stress, the process has long posed problems for Darwinists in that such noisy, predator-attracting and energy-consuming activity appears positively undesirable. However, at the physical level of body function it appears to have a beneficial action on health. In the famous case of Norman Cousins, a programme of self-help involving comedy videos led to a fall in the sedimentation rate of red blood cells (a measure of inflammation) as well as symptom improvement after a bout of laughter. In subsequent, more formal tests, those who listened to a laughter-inducing cassette had a higher threshold for 'pressure-induced' discomfort. Thomas Sydenham, in the 17th century, observed[47] that 'the arrival of a happy clown exercises a more beneficial influence upon the health of a town than twenty asses laden with drugs'. As a physiological phenomenon, laughter may be a complete mystery, but as a preventative or therapeutic medicine it seems effective. Is laughter or CAM more akin to electroconvulsive therapy (ECT)?

MEDICAL IMPERIALISM

Our medicine has become too imperial. Medicine has extended its interest into too many walks of life. It is not so much that we seek preventives or cures that cannot be evidenced, but that we have labelled as therapy anything that may contribute to our well-being. We have become too obsessed with health, concerned that we are a fragile species, when actually we are a remarkably tough one. Health sells. Thomas[48] wrote:

> [H]ealth care has become the new name for medicine. Health-care delivery is what doctors do, along with hospitals and other professionals.... Sooner or later we are bound to get into trouble with this word.... [W]e may be overdoing it, taxing its meaning, to conceal an unmentionable reality that we've somehow agreed not to talk about in public. It won't work. Illness and death still exist and cannot be hidden.

He continues:

> 'Some of the believers among us are convinced ... the country might become a sort of gigantic spa, offering, like the labels of European mineral-water bottles, preventives for everything from weak kidneys to moroseness.'

To this end:[49]

> [C]ommercial announcements are pitches for items to restore failed health: things for stomach gas, constipation, headaches, nervousness, sleeplessness or sleepiness, arthritis, anaemia, disquiet, and the despair of malodorousness, sweat, yellowed teeth, dandruff, furuncles, piles.... Chewing gum is sold as tooth cleanser. Vitamins have taken the place of prayer.... Tennis is a rigorous discipline, a form

> of collective physiotherapy. Jogging is done by swarms of people, out onto the streets each day in underpants, moving in a stolid sort of rapid trudge, hoping by this to stay alive.... Diets mostly for the improvement of everything.

Where does Thomas's protest against our obsession with health relate to CAM? Much CAM is part of this fundamentally unhealthy obsession with health – the idea that health is an end in itself, like the miser's pile of gold. Health requires active promotion and money. Read the magazine's health columns (always ending with 'if you ... seek professional advice'); get a check-up; go on a diet; meditate; jog; take two tablets with water; *Spring* water.

IN CONCLUSION

Science is the key to modern culture. It has changed the world we live in, almost beyond recognition. For some people it may seem as if science has lost sight of our humanity as its enterprises go beyond our understanding. Who really understands a microchip or gene therapy, even in principle, other than the experts themselves? The temptation to disengage and indulge in a soft scientistic, yet profoundly anti-science posture is attractive to some: a world where we may feel that we have better control because we appear to have easier understanding. The task of the humanities is to echo and interpret the concerns arising from scientific advance as they impact on the daily lives – and health – of ordinary people critically and sympathetically, not to retreat to the comforts of attractive irrationality. Our stories illustrate that undergoing treatment is often uncomfortable and demanding. Jake could not tolerate any more and tried to run away from it; Liz entered a world of anxious women, found the prospect of students hard to bear and fainted with the treatment itself; Jen found facing her own illness as well as Geoff's a source of despondency. Modern medicine is not an easy choice. Illness and death will always be with us, as Thomas reminds us. The need to understand the human dimension that our stories illustrate remains as true as ever it did before the rise of science. We dwell in our culture and traditions, take comfort from them and enrich our lives with them – not always rationally. So we may conclude that implausible systems like homeopathy may even have a useful complementary role if understood as personal adjuncts to health and recovery from illness. Interventions that help particular individuals may indeed be alternative (where does orthodox cognitive behavioural therapy overlap with good neighbourliness?) especially outside the publicly funded healthcare system. On the other hand, CAM may be dangerous as an alternative to required orthodoxy and an expensive distraction from health maintenance. Like much modern orthodox medicine this may be especially true when seen in the context of the needs of society and a world full of hunger, poverty and disease.

REFERENCES

1 Myers P. Alternative cure 'zealot' jailed for daughter's death. *The Guardian*. Saturday 6 November; 1993.

2 Ward S. Father who let his diabetic daughter die gets jail term. *The Independent*. Saturday 6 November; 1993.

3 Guthrie D. *A History of Medicine*. Edinburgh: Nelson; 1945.

4 Glymour C, Stalker D. Engineers, cranks, physicians, magicians. *New Engl J Med*. 1983; **308**: 960–4.

5 Thomas L. *The Youngest Science*. Oxford: OUP; 1984.

6 Hoffman D. *The Elements of Herbalism*. Shaftesbury, Dorset: Element Books; 1990.

7 Pietroni P. The meaning of illness: holism dissected. *J Roy Soc Med*. 1987; **80**: 357–60.

8 Thomas K. *Religion and the Decline of Magic*. Harmondsworth: Peregrine, Penguin Books; 1971.

9 Thomas K, op. cit. p. 250.

10 Thomas K. op. cit. p. 268.

11 Whorton JC. Traditions of folk medicine in America. *JAMA*. 1987; **257**: 1632–5.

12 Haller J. Kindly medicines: a history of physio-medicals in American Medicine. *NY State J Med*. 1993; **93**: 133–41.

13 Pickstone JV. Establishment and dissent in nineteenth century medicine: an exploration of some correspondence and connections between religious and medical belief-systems in early industrial England. In: WJ Shiels, editor. *The Church and Healing: studies in church history*. Vol. 19. Oxford: Blackwell; 1982, p. 176.

14 Guthrie D. op. cit. p. 218. *See also*: Neubauer J. Dr John Brown (1735–88) and German Romanticism. *J Hist Ideas*. 1967; **28**: 367–82.

15 Letter from Goethe to Schiller, 19 March 1802.

16 Gevitz N. Sectarian medicine. *JAMA*. 1987; **257**: 1636–40.

17 Gevitz N. op. cit.

18 Standen CS. The implications of the Osteopaths Act: *Complementary Therapies in Medicine* 1993; **1**: 208–10.

19 Young JH. The paradise of quacks. *NY State J Med*. 1993; **93**: 127–33.

20 Whorton JC. op. cit.

21 Georg Ernst Stahl (1659–1734) graduated in medicine from Jena. He went on to profess an animistic system opposed to the materialism of (for example) Boerhaave. His animistic ('a soul which thinks') ideas were developed in his *Theoria medica vera* (1707) – that the soul controls the function and structure of the body, for example, in breathing. His theory opposed the interpretation of human physiology in mechanistic or chemical terms. Pietism was a movement within Lutheranism, with a strong emphasis on biblical study and the devotional life and to its practical consequences in good works. Halle, where Stahl taught at the university, was a leading centre of the pietistic movement. (German Pietism had major influences upon John Wesley, founder of the Methodist movement.)

22 Ranger T. Medical science and Pentecost: the dilemma of Anglicanism in Africa. In: WJ Shiels, editor. *The Church and Healing: studies in church history*. Vol. 19. Oxford: Blackwell; 1982. p. 333–66.

23 Pickstone JV. op. cit.

24 Smith T. Alternative medicine, *BMJ*. 1983; **287**: 307.

25 Wheen F. *How Mumbo Jumbo Conquered the World*. London: Harper Perennial; 2004. p. 129.
26 Hamblin T. More fun in Holy Writ. *BMJ*. 1989; **299**: 1041–2.
27 Sampson WJ. AIDS fraud, finances, and fringes. *NY State J Med*. 1993; **93**: 92–6.
28 *The Guardian*. 13 September; 2008.
29 *The Guardian*. Saturday 8 August; 2004.
30 Pietroni P. op. cit.
31 Pelletier KR. *Holistic Medicine: from stress to optimum health*. New York: Dell Publishing Co; 1979.
32 In a celebrated passage, he writes: 'I am not only lodged in my body as a pilot in a vessel, but that I am besides so intimately conjoined, and as it were intermixed with it, that my mind and body compose a certain unity.' Meditation Six. See: Descartes R. *A Discourse On Method, Meditations On the First Philosophy, and Principles Of Philosophy*. (Trans. John Veitch). Dent, London: Everyman's Library; 1912. For detailed discussion on Descartes' view on the mind–body relation, *see*: Cottingham J. *Descartes*. Oxford: Blackwell; 1986. chapter 5; William B. *Descartes. The Project of Pure Enquiry*. London: Penguin Books; 1978. chapter 10.
33 Smuts JC. *Holism and Evolution*. London: Macmillan; 1926.
34 Poynton JC. Smuts' holism and evolution sixty years on. *Transactions Roy Soc. South Africa*. 1987; **46**: 181–9.
35 Brandon RN. Holism in the philosophy of biology. In: C Glymour and D Stalker, editors. *Examining Holistic Medicine*. Buffalo, NY: Prometheus Books;1985. pp. 127–46.
36 Polanyi M. *Personal Knowledge*. London: Routledge and Kegan Paul; 1958, p. 35.
37 Brandon RN. op. cit.
38 Bunge M. Levels and reduction. *Am J Physiology*. 1977; R75–R82.
39 Hull DL. Reduction and genetics. *J Med Philosophy*. 1981; **6**: 125–43.
40 Zucker A. Holism and reductionism: a view from genetics. *J Med Philosophy*. 1981; **6**: 145–63.
41 Porter R. *The Greatest Benefit to Mankind*. London: Harper Collins; 1977. p. 437. ('Herr Doctor Pettenkofer presents his compliments to Herr Doctor Professor Koch and thanks him for the flask containing the so-called cholera vibrios, which he was kind enough to send. Herr Doctor Pettenkofer has now drunk the entire contents and is happy to be able to inform Herr Doctor Professor Koch that he remains in his usual good health.')
42 Clark A. Psychological causation and the concept of psychosomatic disease. In: C Glymour and D Stalker, editors. *Examining Holistic Medicine*. Buffalo, NY: Prometheus Books; pp. 67–106.
43 Asher R. *Talking Sense*. London: Pitman; 1972.
44 Minerva. *BMJ*. 2010; **341**: 156 reporting on: *Psychosomatic Medicine*. 2010; **72**: 354–6.
45 Minerva. *BMJ*. 2010; **341**: 786 reporting on: *Cancer*. 2010; **116**: 3924–33.
46 Greenfield S. *The Private Life of the Brain*. London: Penguin Books; 2000. p. 153.
47 Greenfield S. op. cit. p. 153.
48 Thomas L. Your very good health. *New Engl J Med*. 1972; **287**: 761–2.
49 Thomas L. The health-care system. *New Engl J Med*. 1975; **293**: 1245–6.

9

Boldness and temperance in treatment

ROLF AHLZÉN

INTRODUCTION

Medical historians describe medical treatment in the late 18th century and in the early 19th as challenging and problematic.[1] The expectations for successful results grew as the sciences progressed. In a few places, such as in post-Revolutionary Paris, there were early signs of a clinical medicine based on firmer scientific foundations. However, doctors still tended to rely on medical traditions that did not meet the challenges of the day. When, for example, cholera rolled over Europe in repeated waves in the early 19th century, most doctors were helpless. No wonder there was room for challengers, for charismatic men driven by their grand theories. Franz Mesmer was one of them. His 'animal magnetism' for a short time triumphed over 'school medicine'. But with his defiance of the medical authorities, Mesmer was bound to get into trouble. His enemies were strong. He was driven away from Vienna, Austria, and then from Paris. Mesmer remained an odd parenthesis in medical history.

In Per-Olof Enquist's novel *The Magnetist's Fifth Winter*, Mesmer, on flight from his enemies in Germany and France, comes to a small Scandinavian town.[2] Here, the daughter of the town physician suffers from blindness and the reason, it seems, may be linked to the way that she lost her mother as a very small girl – that is, she possibly suffered from what would later be called 'hysterical blindness'. Mesmer sees this, and, with the very reluctant acceptance of the father, uses his charismatic power to heal her, using the myth of magnetic fluid permeating cosmos. In the process she becomes deeply emotionally dependent on him.

It remains obscure as to whether Mesmer has used his power over the young woman for healing alone. Mesmer is bold, or even ruthless, with total confidence in his ways of healing. But does he handle this power with temperance, so that he does not infringe on his patients or make them the objects of his desires?

Mesmer uses what we may call 'a healing myth': that of a universal power ('magnetism') permeating cosmos, which he can concentrate as a healing force. He is strongly charismatic; he heals by a combination of hypnosis, trust, attraction and hope. He has, it seems, no second thoughts about his power to bind his patients to himself. Mesmer knew what Michael Balint was to tell GPs in London 250 years later: 'The doctor is the pill;' however, in contrast to the GPs, Mesmer uses this power without any restraint.[3]

This situation may seem to be the very opposite of modern, scientifically based, medicine, where the physician is said to act as the expert in the service of an autonomous, rational patient, applying biomedical and technical skills. The physician of today is supposed to take a sceptical attitude in relation to treatment outcomes, the sound scepticism that systematic empirical knowledge demands. And while Mesmer is applying his healing 'myth' to the young woman and simultaneously attaching her to him, the modern physician relies on empirical methods and clinical detachment. What is regarded as evidence is the result of a sequence of experimentally based investigations, according to procedures that are accepted in a community of scientifically trained persons. There is no longer any room for personal invention or intuition on the part of the clinician.

However, the real-life clinical situation is far more complex than this. Mesmer employs the age old technique of charismatic healing, with its dangers and side effects but also with its strength and its potential for healing. He has one 'grand theory', a myth if we like, which he uses with total dedication. When the physician of the 21st century encounters his or her patient, he or she relies on a 'messy' mixture of personal life experiences, biomedically defined knowledge and practical skills in order to reach diagnoses and to choose treatment. The physician has to intervene in his or her patients' lives, sometimes in ways that are risky, in order to reduce or take away the threat from the disease. However, he or she relies on and is restricted by scientific knowledge, which is one basis for action. The other basis for actions is 'tried experience'. He or she must act, sometimes quite quickly, and he or she has powerful tools for doing this and is also trained to do it.

This preparedness to act may give medical practice an air of confident boldness. This boldness ought to be tempered by restraint. It may, however, free itself from this restraint on occasions, and then lose contact with the ethical foundations of all medical practice. Boldness may then brush temperance and moderation aside. The physician may respond to a technological imperative that has cut its connections to the core values of medical practice.[4]

A DELICATE BALANCE

Let us hold for a while the idea of the bold practitioner. A bold medical practitioner is not the same, of course, as a bold medical researcher. The clinician treats illnesses in human beings. The researcher looks for patterns and regularities in the functions and malfunctions of the body and how different treatments may affect these. Boldness in research may be both important and rewarding, as long as fundamental values of research ethics are respected. Boldness in clinical practice pushes treatments further, is disinclined to stop, and it treats rather than abstains from treatment. The bold clinician tends to take risks also on behalf of his or her patients, in order to potentially win more. New methods fascinate him, and are assumed to be effective. A spirit of curiosity and audacity permeates his or her practice.

The sceptical practitioner, on the other hand, doubts the scope of medical power, is aware of past mistakes and entertains a deep sense of the uncertainty of human knowledge in general and medical knowledge in particular. The sceptical practitioner exercises restraint and temperance in adopting new methods, is unwilling to involve patients in invasive and disrupting treatments with uncertain outcomes and constantly asks whether treatment is really any better than non-treatment.

Of course, these attitudes are not mutually exclusive. Most practitioners hold a combination of both – a fact to which I will return at the end of this chapter. However, there are interesting and relevant differences of emphasis that have far-reaching consequences for medical practice and for the development of medicine in general. The triumphs of scientific medicine during the last century have tended to encourage the boldness I describe, while therapeutic restraint associated with a pessimistic view of outcomes has been pushed into the background.

Still, the delicate balancing between being bold and pushing the limits, for the individual patient and for groups of patients, on the one hand, and moderation and scepticism, on the other, is nothing specific to the physician of the 21st century. The first lines of the Hippocratic *Aphorisms* bear witness to this: 'Life is short, and Art long; the crisis fleeting; experience perilous, and decision difficult.'[5] These words may be read as an invitation to humility and moderation. Throughout history, physicians have been given power, by individuals and by society. They have handled this in very different ways. The 17th-century physicians of playwright and actor Molière (Jean-Baptiste Poquelin) were not able to stop at the right time; they became obsessed with their own power (or perhaps rather desperate about their lack of power).[6]

When there is no favourable response to treatment, the stakes get higher and higher. When the patient finally dies, the death is said to have occurred in spite of the treatments. The fact that bloodletting could persist for centuries as a true panacea must have been due to an unquestioning belief in the healer's methods, regardless of whether these methods were efficient, indifferent or harmful. If a patient died after 300–500 ml of blood had been taken out, it was said to be in spite of, not because of, the treatment. This trust in the healer as the interpreter of the true meaning of the dogma, dictated the treatment and held sway in spite of numerous individual treatment failures. Without comparative studies of different treatments for different conditions, employing statistical means, there was no way of knowing the truth about the outcomes.[7]

When, in the middle of the nineteenth century, medicine finally started integrating the new sciences on a broad scale, new options appeared. The breakthroughs in bacteriology, biochemistry and biophysics seemed to confirm the value of a bold attitude to medicine – in research and in practice. Just as autopsies four centuries earlier had literally opened up new insights into the hidden inside of the dead human body, there now appeared ways of looking into the living body with X-rays, electrocardiograms (ECGs) and the analysis of blood. In Thomas Mann's *The Magic Mountain,* Hans Castorp, the young protagonist, has come to the sanatorium with his sick cousin, and while there he is suspected of also being infected with the tubercle bacillus. In one fascinating scene, Hans undergoes a chest X-ray and afterwards he is shown the mysterious pictures where the lungs appear as vague contours in which the disease may be seen as rounded areas of increased whiteness, if it is there at all. This is an elegant play with the magic of the time, the fascination with the new technology and its ambiguous relation to our everyday bodily being.

Temperance was not easy in the midst of such wonders. Success breeds success and clinical medicine entered into what James Le Fanu calls the era of great victories.[8] He somewhat arbitrarily places this era between about 1935 up until the mid-1970s. One 'bold' breakthrough, which occurred before this period, and took the lives of some dozens of dogs, came in 1921–22, when Banting and Best in Toronto finally pinned down the role of insulin and its relation to the pancreas and to diabetes. The result was a treatment that totally changed the prospects for people with a common and lethal disorder: diabetes mellitus. After insulin came cortisone, penicillin, the psychopharmacological revolution in the mid-1960s, the dialysis machine, the respirator, transplantations and endoscopies. These and other methods were the result of an intimate interplay between clinical observations, basic research and applied research. They thrived in a climate of optimism and daring – and, it must be conceded, the relative absence of ethical restrictions. As Le Fanu writes:

> If clinical science was to progress it certainly could not put internal constraints on itself but must be capable of pushing at the boundaries of the technically feasible.[9]

Clinical boldness and scientific optimism went hand in hand in a mutually reinforcing symbiosis. As long as the victories were impressive in the eyes of most people and as long as the abuse of power did not become too obvious there was not much critique against the tendency to push the limits further.

PUSHING THE LIMITS IN PSYCHIATRY

However, there was one area where substantial success was still absent, an area where the general atmosphere was one of pessimism rather than optimism: psychiatry. The expectations born in the 1880s, with the advent of bacteriology, had also reached the young science of psychiatry. As paralysie générale was shown to be caused by the syphilis spirochete in its fourth stage of infection, analogies were not surprisingly made to other major psychiatric diseases like schizophrenia (Kraepelin's dementia praecox). However, bacteriology, it would soon turn out, was not the answer to the riddle of psychiatric disease. Europe went into the era of large psychiatric institutions without any established remedies for the conditions that were the reason why people were confined there.

The great asylums of the first half of the 20th century were places where long baths, spinning chairs and locking-in belts were measures of control rather than treatment. So while the rest of the medical scene was in a phase of rapid progress, psychiatry was confined to methods that had progressed no further than the detention of insane people. Freud's talking cure was certainly not for those tens of thousands of more or less chronic patients who inhabited the asylums.[10]

It is not surprising that in this climate dreams thrived of more efficient, more 'scientific', methods. These hopes were of course inspired by what went on in so-called somatic medicine. If diabetes could be successfully treated with insulin injections, and if mental illnesses are dysfunctions of the brain, there must surely be similar methods, based on more or less knowledge about the brain, that may alter its way of functioning and hence mean a relief from psychiatric symptoms. The psychiatrists were not so much bold as eager – eager to do something for their patients, to consolidate their own professional status and to make the conditions of the asylum acceptable. This was the general background to the introduction of three methods in psychiatry, of which two would be discarded – while the third would survive, although in a radically modified way.

The history is illuminating in several ways, not least because it gives us a hint of how unexpected observations may lead to new therapeutic strategies. It had been noted that patients with diabetes who also happened to suffer from psychiatric illness and who went into a short insulin coma – that must have been rather common given the often unclean preparation of insulin at the time and the difficulties of good surveillance of blood glucose levels[11] – seemed to get some relief from their psychiatric symptoms. The inference was obvious: the very low blood glucose level must have a positive effect on the brain. The mechanism was, of course, totally mysterious, just as the brain mechanisms behind psychiatric diseases were unknown. It was a classic 'black box situation': an input, the insulin injections, leading to the coma, led to a result, the amelioration of symptoms.

Insulin coma was introduced in the 1930s and it was used for at least 20 years in the treatment of several psychiatric illnesses. It was regarded as the only specific treatment for schizophrenia. Manfred Sakel in Vienna developed it from animal tests to humans, despite a widespread fear of the risks associated with the method. The preparations were extensive, the protracted treatment took place in certain specialised units and convulsions and other somatic reactions were very common.[12] Many patients emerged from therapy periods as grossly obese, the mortality was relatively high and brain damage occurred in some cases. In spite of these serious problems with the method it was seen as a success: 'All references, particularly the comments of doctors on the atmosphere in insulin units, describe tremendous enthusiasm.'[13] In the early 1950s, about the same time as frontal lobotomy came into disrepute, and with the arrival of the neuroleptics, marked by chlorpromazine (Hibernale) in 1953–54, it went into oblivion, after several studies had questioned its specific effect on schizophrenia.

The similarities to another psychiatric treatment developed during this period are obvious. When Egas Moniz in 1949 received the Nobel Prize in 'physiology' (that is, in what we today call medicine) it was because of his application of the experiences from a very strange case from the late 19th century, where Nicholas Cage, an American railway worker, suffered a terrible accident. A metal splint passed through the orbita penetrating his forebrain, cutting off some connections between the frontal cortex and the rest of the brain. Cage survived, but he was changed from a decent and loyal worker and husband into an indifferent and morally dubious man.[14] The case, thought Moniz, seemed to indicate that if the connections from frontal areas to the rest of the brain were cut, the resulting change of personality would go in the direction of increased calmness and of freedom from anguish and other strong emotions.

Interestingly enough, the Swiss physician Gottlieb Burckhardt had performed psychosurgical interventions already in 1888. Burckhardt's clinical experiments, however, were received with disregard, and he gave the idea up. When professor of neurology Moniz took it up in the early 1930s, it was on the basis of an idea common at the time: that psychiatric disease had its origin in disorders of the synapses.[15] He relied on the results of experiments conducted on chimpanzees at the time, and made the conclusion that it was necessary to

> change the synaptic facilities and also the path that is chosen by the stimuli in their continuous process, in order to change the corresponding thoughts and to force them into other channels. For this reason … I decided to cut the connecting fibres of the neurons concerned.[16]

Frontal lobotomy was introduced on a broad scale in many countries and was generally thought of as successful. The Nobel Prize is an indication of this. Even when it became obvious that the people who had undergone it were often radically transformed in their personality, developing indifference verging on that of a 'zombie' ... even then it continued. The last frontal lobotomy in Sweden was performed in 1964. As with insulin coma therapy, the disappearance seems to be a combined result of accumulated insights into both the practical and ethical problems of the treatment, along with the advent of the neuroleptics.[17]

Was lobotomy a 'desperate treatment', deeply unethical by today's standards? It is far too easy to pass judgements and to condemn the practices of a time where values and possibilities were so different. It must be understood that the patients undergoing lobotomy were very ill, and often dangerous to themselves and/or others. What else was there to offer these patients? Nevertheless, the irreversibility of the measure and its mutilating character may have been expected to curb its application on a broad scale. This was not the case. Psychiatry needed breakthroughs, and humanitarian considerations were contaminated by professional ambition and the needs for social control. Internal and external influences were strong. What chances were there of temperance in a difficult situation like this?

The third of the bold attempts to treat psychiatric illness was electroconvulsive therapy (ECT). The idea to electrically induce seizures had a similar origin as insulin coma treatment: random observations that some psychiatric patients seemed to have a reduction of symptoms after epileptic seizures. In the early 1930s, Hungarian psychiatrist Ladislaus von Meduna tried the drug Metrazol to induce seizures in schizophrenic patients, and later, with more success, in people with deep depressions. Some years later, Italian researchers Ugo Cerletti and Lucio Bini started using electricity for what was at the time called 'electro shock therapy'. Knowledge of the new method spread rapidly. The first treatment was given in the United States in 1939, and it became popular and widespread in the 1940s and 1950s in many countries, before going into what was probably a temporary decline in the 1970s and 1980s.[18]

In Ken Kesey's *One Flew Over the Cuckoo's Nest* from 1963, the main character, McMurphy, is pacified by means of repeated convulsive treatments.[19] Milos Forman engraved this image of ECT into the heads of those millions who saw his film with the same name. When, in the 1970s and 1980s, the treatment was modified, when the patient was given narcosis and muscle relaxation and the seizures reduced to a minimum – it was almost impossible to achieve a re-evaluation of this treatment, despite evidence for its efficiency. Only in recent years has ECT become what the early pioneers for it hoped it would be – a serious and respected alternative, or sometimes complement, to drugs and psychotherapy for situations of severe depressive disorders. When used with temperance, this once so 'bold', sometimes coercive and perhaps even desperate, treatment is now generally thought of as a valuable part of the arsenal of evidence-based psychiatric treatments.

RESTRAINT IN A TECHNOLOGICAL ERA

Medicine historically seems to have risked pushing the limits of treatment without sufficient restraint in two principally different situations: first, when there has been a major breakthrough in some area of the basic biomedical sciences and when very promising clinical applications (sometimes associated with chances of great economic profits) appear and, second, when there have been no breakthroughs at all, but the human needs for remedies are still very urgent. The latter was the case with psychiatry in the early 20th century.

But who, then, was 'bold', in the sense that I have used this word? The researcher who attempted to develop new lines of therapy? The physician who against historically bad odds ventured into a new area of treatment, where the results were at best uncertain? Or the patient who consented to undergo the treatment? Did informed consent actually occur? In the case of psychiatric treatment, the patients were often considered to be incompetent. Paternalism reigned. It was within the physician's power to choose treatment and the restraints, whether on the side of the patient or from society, were weak.

This is of course not only the case for psychiatric medicine. On the somatic side, clinical research was conducted that would stand no chance of being accepted today. One example was a Swedish caries research project, conducted in Lund from 1951–55, where a group of young men with severe mental retardation were, without informed consent, given a very sweet and sticky fudge. They could eat as much as they wanted and they had their mouths full of sugar much of the time. Meticulous surveillance was made of pH in the mouth, bacterial plaques on the teeth, flow of saliva – and of the brisk appearance of dental caries and periodontitis.

It is generally agreed that the information from this project on how dental caries develop and what may protect them was vital to the successful preventive strategies of the coming decades. But was this research ever tempered by awareness of the rights of the non-consenting research subjects? It rather seems as if the researchers followed the tradition of bold research, where the findings would more than compensate for the comparatively limited harm that may have been inflicted on a group of people.[20]

But this particular form of boldness was to be checked. It did not survive the reflection on the experiences of the Second World War, particularly those of the Nazi physicians' experiments. Neither did it survive the increased emphasis on individual choice and the gradual weakening of traditional belief in authority. The constraints imposed by research ethics were the first to be spelled out in declarations and codes (the most authoritative being the Declaration of Helsinki), but clinical practice followed soon after. Autonomy became the order of the day. The idea of a personal right to self-determination was seen as an outcome from ideas of personal rights, regardless of possible risks, but also as a way of protecting patients against what was increasingly thought to be dangers inherent in the medical technological development. For even if insulin coma and ECT therapy had obvious delicate ethical implications, these could be seen as relatively minor to those that appeared when respirators, dialysis machines, full parenteral nutrition and transplantation techniques appeared.

The physician as the cruel imposer of life-sustaining measures on patients that really should have the right to die … this image became widespread. If physicians during most of human history were faced with the dilemma of having too few tools for interventions, they now had an abundance of possibilities, the use of which could be deeply problematic. For the physician of the late 20th century, moderation in the face of multiple technological options was becoming an even greater challenge than the relative powerlessness of colleagues in earlier centuries.

New actors appeared on the scene. As historian David Rothman shows in his *Strangers At the Bedside,* there was no general trust that physicians would be able to self-regulate, given these new tools of power.[21] Restraint would have to come from somewhere else. From about 1970, there was a series of legal processes in the United States, where lawyers appeared as 'strangers at the bedside', demanding a say on what earlier were seen as exclusively medical decisions. The European countries got their fare share of this but, for historical and constitutional reasons, not to the same extent as was the case in the United States. Not only were lawyers engaged in the struggle against medical hegemony: they were joined by ethicists and patient organisations. In this process, physicians were not dethroned but they were certainly pushed out of a position of total and unquestioned control. It is not unreasonable to look upon the rise of medical ethics in this context. If, and only if, the medical profession could prove itself capable of dealing with these new tools in an acceptable way, would it be able to defend its position as master of life and death. The formal development of medical ethics was one central answer to this.

Most of the ethical discussion focused on the challenges that high technology medicine posed. But the professional ethos of physicians is one and the same. The physician of the intensive care unit acts from the same moral position as do his or her colleagues in the rural health centre, or the psychiatric clinic or the neonatal unit: 'Sometimes cure, often ameliorate, always console.'[22] This points to the other side of the coin, where diseases are stronger than the human efforts to curb them. The developments in medicine not only gave new options for life-sustaining treatments where there earlier had been few or no chances; it also meant that new possibilities for palliation appeared.

The dividing point between a situation where most efforts are aiming at cure and the patient herself or himself hopes for this, and a situation where hopes for cure have gone … this shift of perspective proved to be very difficult, at least in some situations. This decision is certainly not made easily and hardly without experience and training. It involves adopting another position, a new set of goals, for the measures taken. The physician, so used to seeing himself or herself as the one who protects and prolongs life, is now the one who has the responsibility to improve the ill person's quality of life prior to death. For some physicians this was not difficult, as they saw it as just an extension of their basic task: to ameliorate and console. For others it was far more difficult. Physician and patient may clash, or the ill person may just not be able to present his or her 'authentic' desires. And the complexity of the task was of course increased by the presence of other people who rightly asked for influence: close relatives and, in some countries, also lawyers and courts.

Palliation requires what I have here called temperance, in making the decision to give up the goal of cure and in balancing the patient's different needs during the period when the disease runs its course and death approaches. But one may also say that boldness is involved here – that is, the courage on the part of the responsible physician to bring the question up at the right moment and then find the appropriate way to discuss it with his or her patient. This is a different kind of audacity than that required for swift action or aggressive treatment. It requires that finely tuned perception that Kathryn Montgomery writes about as 'clinical judgement' – an amalgamation of biomedical knowledge, practical skills, imagination and self-knowledge.[23] The same capacity must be present if the patient is not competent to take decisions. Facing this situation, the physician will need boldness and temperance intertwined into a unity of well-balanced judgement.

Is the physician of the early 21st century generally incapable of stopping life-sustaining treatments in time? Is she or he the helpless prisoner of the utopian aspirations of a profession that sees death as the ultimate failure? This is the general impression one could easily get from two or three decades of debate around 'end-of-life' decisions. But the support for this in research is weak. In Örebro, in Sweden, ethics researcher Mia Svantesson interviewed nurses and physicians in intensive care units for their experiences and positions on matters of withdrawal of treatment or abstention from treatment.[24] The picture that emerges is certainly not that of a radical gulf between the two professions, rather that of caution and … yes, moderation and temperance. The same impression is given in Sören Holm's interviews with nurses and physicians in Denmark about their reflections on moral dilemmas that they encounter in their work.[25] There is certainly not, in these interviews, any 'technological imperative' to be seen – but more the pressures and calamities of hard decisions. There are differences in position between the professional groups, but these are not big. They are larger inside the professions than between them, and they seem to be the result not of basic differences of values but of different perspectives on the clinical situation and, of course, different degrees of final responsibility.

Patient autonomy is a corner stone of modern healthcare systems. It is far more difficult to know the meaning and scope of this right to self-determination. It has rightly been asked whether, for example, an old man on haemodialysis who has had several cerebral thromboses and who is exhausted and low in mood is capable of exerting himself an autonomous and informed choice on the continuation or discontinuation of the dialysis. Questions like these have had a prominent place in the medical ethical debate for the last 20 to 30 years, and it is easy to see that there are few general answers. There seems to be no escape from those messy, 'unclean' decisions where all the particularities of the situation must be recognised and brought to coexist with general ethical values and often also legal restrictions. One may see this as a delicate balancing, as an exceedingly complex act of interpreting a seriously and perhaps terminally ill person's last will in relation to prognosis and dignity of life. Medical facts will appear as background data for such a decision, but the choice is, at the end, solidly within the moral realm. In this, the physician is the one with the final responsibility, but he or she certainly possesses no privileged road to the right judgement.

There are good reasons to doubt whether most physicians feel that they are prepared for such decisions – to the extent that anyone can be prepared for them. There is a striking difference between the weight of such predicaments in a clinician's everyday work, and, on the other hand, the absence of preparation for dealing with them. What is the appropriate answer to this lack of awareness, this relative powerlessness, in the midst of all-powerful medical technology? Any answers to the questions of if, when and how to stop a treatment – or not to start it – are so deeply intertwined with the intricacies of the life worlds of those who need our help, as well as with the uncertainties of diagnosis, treatment and prognosis. The decision is fundamentally ethical and, as such, requires an understanding of the lives of ill people, their lived experiences. Temperate action requires a profound acquaintance with this dimension of the clinical encounter, as well as with the epistemology of nature, of the scientifically described body.

But it is not only the physician who faces the challenge to be both bold and capable of moderation and temperance. The ill person, particularly the seriously ill person, will need courage in order to face the situation. Many ill people struggle with feelings of guilt, and of being overwhelmed with the burdens of a new situation. If they are also expected to take hard decisions on the basis of very limited knowledge of medical matters, it is not difficult to see how evasion and withdrawal may be the most tempting attitude. The principle of autonomy becomes dictatorial if it leads physicians to put too heavy a burden on very ill people close to their death. As Richard Zaner, with great sensitivity, shows in his *Ethics and the Clinical Encounter*, the physician, in cooperation with other professionals in contact with the patient and with close relatives when possible, must attempt to 'reconstruct' the will of the seriously ill patient, when he or she is not able to do this himself or herself.[26] The fact that a person does not object, or is not able to object, or that the relatives hold strong positions on which course to adopt, cannot be enough for taking the decision to start or end life-sustaining measures. Neither can the fact that any such 'reconstruction' is bound to be both uncertain and difficult be reason enough not to make the attempt. With the concepts I have chosen: it is both bold and temperate to take the full responsibility in such a situation and to face the complexity of the decision.

REVIVING VIRTUES

Almost 2400 years after Aristotle formulated the idea of virtue as the balancing between two extremes, we find this balance urgently needed in clinical medicine. Aristotle's focus was on unique actions in complex situations. In the words of Richard Tarnas:

> The proper aim of ethics was not to determine the nature of the absolute virtue, but to be a virtuous person. That task was necessarily complex and ambiguous, evading final definition, and required practical solutions to practical problems rather than absolute principles that were universally true.[27]

Each virtue, then, according to Aristotle is the balance between extremes. My assumption is that clinical action is characterised by *phronesis*, practical wisdom, when the virtues of clinical practice are in balance with one another. Central among Aristotle's virtues are courage and temperance. I here take courage to be basically equivalent to what I have called boldness – the disposition to act swiftly and decisively. Temperance is the countervailing power – that of reflection, scepticism – and if boldness is not there, temperance may result in indecisiveness and passivity.

Of course, this is nothing new for medicine in the 20th and 21st centuries. However, the consequences of *not* striking this balance are more far-reaching and potentially devastating than ever before. Whether it is the treatment of Rachel's diabetes, of Jake's irritable bowel, Liz's cervical pathology or Geoff's depression, the goals of medicine are the same: the reduction of human suffering, the promotion of human dignity and well-being and the giving back of hope and possibilities in life. Only a bold temperance will lead to this goal.

REFERENCES

1 Johannisson K. *Medicinens öga: sjukdom, medicin, samhälle – historiska erfarenheter* [*The Eye of Medicine: Disease, Medicine, Society – Historical Experiences*]. Stockholm: Norstedts; 1990.
2 Enquist P-O. *The Magneticist's Fifth Winter.* London: Quartet Books; 1989.
3 Balint M. *The Doctor, His Patient and the Illness.* London: Pitman; 1964.
4 Reiser S. *Medicine and the Reign of Technology.* Cambridge: Cambridge University Press; 1978.
5 Hippocrates: *The Aphorisms.* Encyclopedia Britannica. Searchword 'Hippocrates'. www.britannica.com/EBchecked/topic/266627/Hippocrates (accessed 13 March 2012).
6 Molière. For example: *Le Malade Imaginaire* or *Tartuffe.* See: *The Moliere Encyclopedia.* Gaines JF, editor. Westport, CT: Greenwood; 2002.
7 The first studies of this sort came in the 1840s, when patients admitted to hospital for pneumonia were grouped in two, where one group of patients got bloodletting and the other not. The latter group did, of course, better, and the difference could be shown to be unlikely to be attributable to a random difference. Seigworth GR. Bloodletting over the centuries. *New York State Journal of Medicine.* 1980; **80**: 2022–8.
8 Le Fanu J. *The Rise and Fall Of Modern Medicine.* London: Abacus; 2000.
9 Ibid., p. 202.
10 In Sweden, the number culminated in about 1960, when it is estimated that about 65 000 people out of a population of about seven million lived in the large psychiatric hospitals. Sjöström B. *Kliniken tar över darskapen: Om den moderna svenska psykiatrins framväxt* [*Insanity moves into the clinic: On the emergence of the modern Swedish psychiatry*]. Göteborg: Daidalos; 1992.
11 We may compare this to Rachel, who in our stories probably will get an insulin pump that continuously monitors the glucose levels and injects exactly the appropriate dose of pure humane insulin.
12 Marti-Ibanez F. *The Great Physiodynamic Therapies In Psychiatry: an historical reappraisal.* New York, NY: Pau B. Hoeber; 1956. pp. 13–75.
13 Jones K. Insulin coma therapy in schizophrenia. *Journal of the Royal Society of Medicine.* 2000; **93**: 147–9.
14 The case is well described and reflected upon in Antonio R. Damasio's *Descarte's Error: emotion, reason, and the human brain.* New York, NY: G.P. Putnam; 1994. pp. 7–12.
15 Gross D, Schaefer G. Egas Moniz (1874-1955) and the 'invention' of modern psychosurgery: a historical and ethical reanalysis under special consideration of Portuguese original sources. *Neurosurgical Focus.* 2011; **30**(2): E8.
16 Ibid.
17 Ogren K, Sandlund M. Psychosurgery in Sweden 1944–1964. *Journal Of the History Of the Neuroscience.* 2005; **14**: 353–67.
18 Lebenson ZM. The history of electroconvulsive treatment in the United States and its place in America: a personal memoir. *Comprehensive Psychiatry.* 1999; **40**: 173–81.
19 Kesey K. *One Flew Over the Cuckoo's Nest.* London: Pan Books; 1983.
20 This so called Vipeholm project has been described and debated in Sweden for several years. With few exceptions, those who have analysed it have found it to be unacceptable in the light of those basic principles for research ethics that would a decade later lead to the adoption of the Helsinki declaration in June 1964. See

Bommenel E. *Sockerförsöket* [*The Sugar Experiment*] [dissertation]. University of Lund; 1996.

21 Rothman D. *Strangers At the Bedside: a history of how law and bioethics transformed medical decision making.* Cambridge: Cambridge University Press; 1991. Chapter 1 in particular.

22 This aphorism is usually ascribed to Hippocrates, but it is nowhere found in the Corpus Hippocraticum. Personal communication from Raimo Puustinen.

23 Montgomery K. *How Doctors Think: clinical judgment and the practice of medicine.* Oxford: Oxford University Press; 2006.

24 Svantesson M. *Postpone Death?: nurse-physician perspectives on life-sustaining treatments and ethics rounds.* Örebro Studies in Medicine; 2008.

25 Holm S. *Ethical Problems in Clinical Practice: the ethical reasoning of health care professionals.* Manchester: Manchester University Press; 1997.

26 Zaner R. *Ethics and the Clinical Encounter.* Englewood Cliffs, NJ: Prentice Hall; 1988.

27 Tarnas R. *The Passion Of the Western Mind: understanding the ideas that have shaped our world view.* London: Pimlico; 1991. p. 67.

Index